Healthy-Licious

RUTH BALSIGER

A SELF-CARE GUIDE TO BRING DELICIOUS BEAUTY,
BALANCE, AND LOVE TO THE MIRACLE THAT IS YOU

Healthy-Licious.

Published in Australia by RB Publishing.

Copyright © 2019 by Ruth Balsiger

To contact the author, visit www.ithriveforhealth.com.au

978-0-6485530-0-7

NATIONAL LIBRARY OF AUSTRALIA · A catalogue record for this book is available from the National Library of Australia

Photography: Chris Bromell

Food photography & styling: Danica Zuks

Acknowledgements:
Thank you to my amazing husband Anthony for believing in me. To my gorgeous daughters for being my inspiration and giving me strength when things go haywire. Thank you to beautiful Bethrene for always being my guardian angel. To everyone who made this incredible journey of mine possible. Thank you for buying this book and helping to make this world a healthier, happier, more radiant place.

Contents

How to Use this Book 5

Foreword 6

Introduction 7

Part 1: Healthy Mind—Healthy Life 9

Self-Compassion 13

Sleep 19

Stress Less 24

Just Breathe! 33

Part 2: Yummy-Licious — A Whole Foods Love Affair 37

Clarifying Food Confusion 41

Abundant Life and Self-Compassionate Weight Loss 50

Cravings and Different Forms of Hunger 57

Overeating & Binge Eating: How Much Is Enough? 67

The Next Generation 77

Let's Get Cooking 84

RECIPES 85

Part 3: Get Moving 129

We Are Born to Move 133

How to Keep Your Healthy Up 147

Weight Loss and Movement 153

Let's Play 157

EXERCISES 160

Conclusion and Moving Forward 165

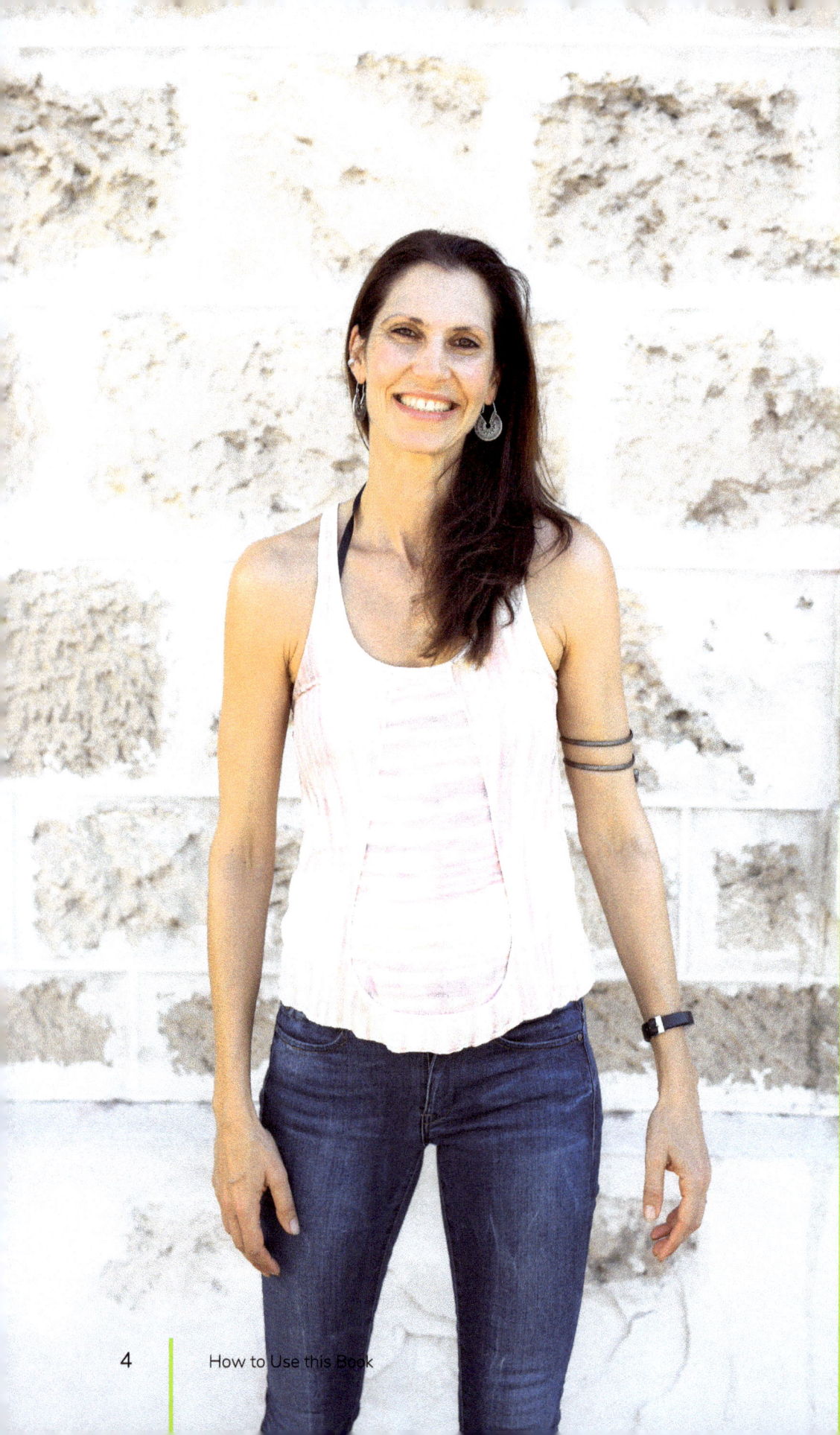

How to Use this Book

How to Use this Book

My goal is to empower and guide you on your journey toward a happier, healthier, more fulfilled and more radiant version of yourself. I will share with you my own experiences that taught me the *truths* laid out in this book. It's important for you to know that you are not alone on this road—I have been there, too. In fact, I am still on this road. It is where I thrive, and it is where I know how to guide you to your greatest personal achievement and life satisfaction.

This book has three parts. In *Part One*, I lay the foundation and make the case for self-care as the essential element for your lifetime success in living a healthy-licious life. It addresses sleep patterns, stress management and meditation. In *Part Two*, I teach you about hunger and satiety, the cues for overeating, and how to be proactive in your children's nutrition. In *Part Three*, I discuss the essential elements of movement and the joy of nurturing a body in motion.

Healthy-Licious is designed so you can jump straight away to any section of any chapter and find the support you need at that particular time of your life. Reading it from top to bottom might not be for you, and that is okay. Your journey is uniquely yours. I want you to find y*our* way of reading **Healthy-Licious** so you can totally get the best out of it for YOU.

Foreword

At the outset, I want you to know that I do not have it all together, all of the time. Like anyone, I am a work in progress and I admit that I battle with perfectionism. The voice in my head argues "I am unworthy." It baits me with lies and turns me from being awesomely in tune with my physical, mental and emotional self into a I-can-numb-this mode.

What always brings me back from those moments of raw insecurity is that I know the truth of who I am. I know that I am a good human being, that I am capable and powerful, kind and considerate, intelligent and diligent and, without sounding egotistical, I know I'm awesome! I empower myself by nourishing my body with yummy-licious wholesome foods, I-can-do-anything moves and healing, and feel-good self-nurturing. I always come back to it.

More times than I can count I have been asked, "How on earth do you manage to keep your healthy up?" "Don't you get bored?" "How do you balance your healthy lifestyle practises with your social life?" I am a business owner, wife, mum of two girls, one pre-teen and one teenager (what on earth was I thinking?! I have no idea how to survive the next 2-3 years without going insane... Can you relate?) How do I fit healthy-licious living into my busy world?

Do you want to know my secrets? The plain truth is that I look after myself. I move my body regularly. I nurture myself with wholesome foods. I exchange self-loathing with kind, compassionate words. I accept myself with grace. I create a warm, loving home for myself (and my family) and I feel whole. Honestly, there is no other place I want to be, no other space I'd rather come back to. No matter how often I might fall in or out, this healthy place in and outside of me is where I am strongest. It is where I best take on the world's adversities, where I feel happiest, and where I glow and grow.

Introduction

Have you ever wondered how life would feel and look if you were living the healthiest, most vibrant, radiant and energised version of yourself? Do you feel confused by conflicting messages about what it takes to become healthy?

Are your efforts to take control met by sabotage? Does your quest for body transformation feel like a punishment? Have you given every last effort to take control of your body and your life, only to fail again and again? Do you feel powerless? Have you abandoned hope of ever feeling comfortable in your own skin? Do you sometimes hate your body?

Well, you are not alone. I relate. I have been there. It is frustrating, confusing, and frankly...can feel hopeless. It does not feel particularly blessed, does it?

But...what if your body is not your enemy, bent on sabotaging your efforts to feel good, to move well and feel content? What if, what is missing in your success story is not about tracking macros, counting calories or punishing yourself with strenuous exercise? In fact, what if healthy living is not achieved by self-loathing, body shaming and disempowering limitations?

Discovering the truth of my own wonder-licious self came at a price. I hope that sharing my story will fast-track your own journey. I hope my experiences will ease your pain and enable you access to your truth. I hope to facilitate a paradigm shift that gives you power to love yourself, your life and your body.

My wake-up call came in my teens. A brain aneurysm gave me newfound appreciation and reverence for not only my body's mind-blowing capacity to heal, to move and to thrive, but also a greater understanding of how critical it is to provide space, nurturing and care for my body to heal, to move and to thrive. The brain surgery gave me an appreciation for my body's ability to move as I directed it. With that experience failed to teach me that it was equally important to feed my body well so that it could perform well. I learnt that through the consequences of dieting and disordered eating. True health is more than being able to move your body in all the right ways. Health requires an abundance mindset (rather than scarcity and restriction) to create a balanced diet bursting with colourful, wholesome foods to bring out the best in you.

I thought this was the secret, but I was actually still missing a crucial piece of understanding. Not until I nearly lost the love of my life did I become fully present to what true, balanced health looks like. Healthy-licious awesomeness cannot exist nor sustain itself in the absence of self-acceptance, self-kindness and self-respect.

I'm not alone in my struggle with this concept. This challenge seems to be the birthright of women. We are masterful at nurturing everybody else, but we find ourselves quite lost when it comes to turning those gifts inward and caring for our own needs. However, dedicating time every day to feeding your soul is an absolutely necessary act of love if you are serious about transforming your own life.

I count myself so lucky and blessed. My journey brought me to this place where I live daily with a wonderful feeling of wholesome radiance. Energy runs through my entire body, my soul, my mind! It fills me with true vitality and makes me jump out of my skin with happy vibrancy! It is a feeling where I know all is well because I am at home in my strong body, my clear mind and my joyful soul! Health is no longer a vague concept where my mind chases a fantasy-type body image through restrictive diets and joyless, punishing workouts.

Instead, health has become for me, an empowered feeling of knowing how to nurture myself with movement that feels good, whole foods that beautify me from the in- and outside, and re-balancing acts of self-care.

This is the wonderful empowerment I want to share with you, my gorgeous reader! The fact is, no matter where you are beginning, regardless of your age, your physical condition, or your past experiences with weight loss, you are in the perfect place to begin. You can fall in love with your most healthy-licious self...and I would be honoured to help you.

Are you ready to change gears and abandon negative self-talk, self-limiting beliefs and self-sabotaging habits that don't serve the best that is within you? Are you ready to embrace all the glory that you are (and always have been)?

It is time. It is time to learn how to nurture your body to bring out the best that is within you. You were born for this. You deserve to be the happiest, most radiant, most gorgeous version of yourself.

All that stands between you and transformation is your decision to take a leap of faith in YOURSELF. Trust yourself to discover what uniquely suits you, in your own way, in your own time, in your own already-over-scheduled lifestyle. You can own the stunning goddess within you! Trust yourself. Trust me. There is truly no better feeling than coming home to your best self! I know how to lead you there.

PART 1:

HEALTHY MIND — HEALTHY LIFE

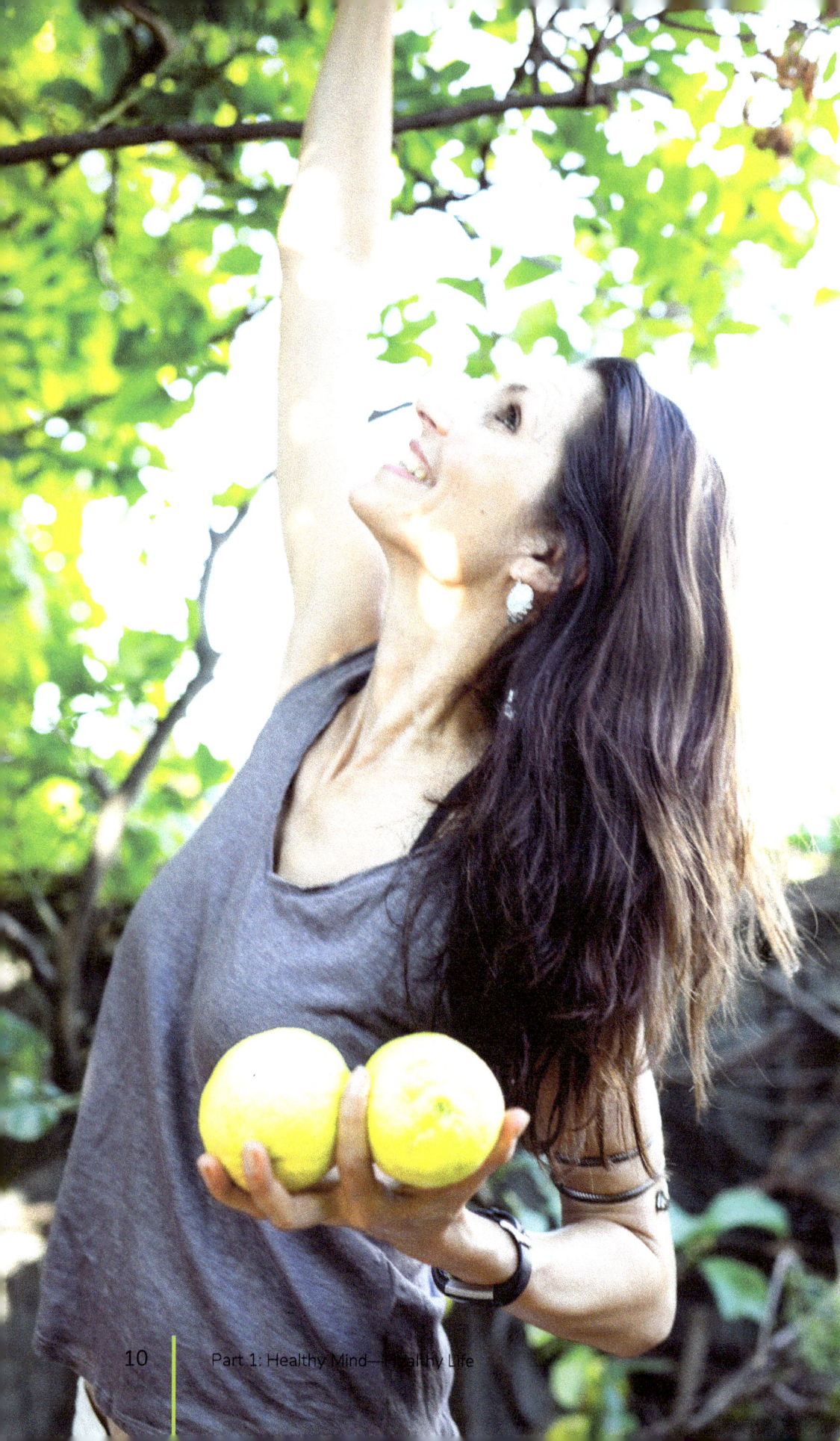

| Part 1: Healthy Mind—Healthy Life

My Own Story

September 2019 will mark nine years into a new journey I embarked on with my husband. We took our two beautiful little baby girls, aged 2 and 4 at that time, on an exciting adventure across the world from Switzerland to Australia. I remember my first impressions as I stepped outside the airport and took in the stunning wildness. The air was cool; night had fallen and the sky sang with the strange music of foreign birds. Perth, Western Australia, intrigued me. To me, it was the most bizarre cross between a modern city and a laid-back rural village.

What began as a crazy holiday adventure abruptly became our new day-to-day reality. My husband was offered permanent employment, so we decided to stay and settle in Perth. I was suddenly now living on the other side of the world with two little girls who neither knew nor understood a word of English. Excitement quickly morphed into shock and fear. Everything was different. I was very clearly a European alien in a new and foreign land. Some of the school mums stared at me in disbelief: "You are walking? You're not driving?" They looked at me like I had lost all my senses; I let them belittle me with their different ways of thinking.

But I had no time for being scared or puzzled. I had to make things work, and **fast**. Miya (my 4-year old) needed to start school, and I needed to furnish a house. I had to learn about all the big and little things that make the Australian world go 'round.

With all I had, I threw myself head-first into this new life. I put my nutrition studies on hold, became a personal trainer and started my own business.

I worked to keep up with all the new customs and traditions, the English language and the many unspoken rules. I poured my heart and soul into my business, did further studies to add on qualifications to shape it into what I needed it to be. I became qualified as a Wellness Coach, as a Health Coach and as a Nutrition Coach, all whilst being the best I could be as my daughters' mum and my husband's wife.

Along the way, though, I somehow forgot about caring for and nurturing myself. I was so busy with everyone else's needs and making our new life work that I totally excluded myself from the equation. Until one morning...I woke up with my relationship in pieces.

My husband had started living a different life, one far more exciting than the boring life I was living. His world had become all about work and the after-work parties which entailed alcohol, sexy young women and staying out until dawn. Somewhere in my ambition to make our new existence awesome, I had lost myself, and we had lost each other. I was heart-broken and felt betrayed.

The hard truth was that my deepest betrayal was mine. I had not nurtured myself. I had not paused to breathe and recharge my batteries. I had not listened to my needs, my desires, to all that makes me who I am. I would like to address here that I am a deeply spiritual person. I believe that we all have come here with a purpose—that every step we take and every decision we make propels us forward to where we need to be in order to fulfil our missions. Sometimes this journey can have lots of detours, especially if we forget to take breaks to listen to our hearts and to what is important to us—to our values, our desires and to what makes me "me" or you "you."

Well, I decided to go on the search for myself again and back to what I believe in, which is true holistic health—this includes the needs of my soul and my mind. I am also a bit of a stubborn, romantic soul and not one to give up easily. I believe that true love is worth fighting for. So, I needed to find out whether my husband, the love of my life, felt the same about me and about "us." He did. So, the search for myself led me also to a much more beautiful, strong and authentic version of "us."

This experience taught me (rather unkindly) how important self-nurture is for true health. Somehow, we women hold on to the belief that self-nurture is something very egoistic, so we don't do it. We are exceptionally wonderful at nurturing everyone else around us, but we often neglect ourselves.

I invite you to challenge those thoughts. Turn them around. What if denying yourself the care that your body and soul hunger for is actually being selfish—not the other way around? If you are tuning out from what your body needs, what your heart desires, what your soul knows deeply to be true because you think that it is not your time to live and thrive, you are denying the world the glory of your full potential. You are short-changing yourself (and everyone who matters to you) the beauty of living in a world blessed by the expression of your life's mission. Can you see how very selfish this is? We owe this world the beauty that flows through each of us as a nourished soul, mind and body. The light and glow we can individually and collectively bring to bear will cause our world to be happier, healthier and far more wonderful than we can conceive in our wildest dreams.

Self-Compassion

THE MISSING LINK

What does self-compassion have to do with being healthy? My answer is "Everything!" I have learnt the hard way and have seen the lesson repeated in the lives of many of my clients and students. Without the ability to love yourself, it is virtually impossible to give your body, mind and spirit the care and nurture that these parts of you deserve. Only when you accept and respect yourself can you open the door to the incredible beauty of a deeply connected mind, body and soul. It is an experience that will blow your mind, and not because you have convinced yourself that you are the greatest person to walk the planet. Instead, you will come to a place of deeply knowing that you are enough just as you are. No matter your place in your journey, you are **love**. You are **beauty**. **You** are worth living your best, most radiant and vibrant life.

True health and well-being can only come from a place of self-compassion. Self-compassion, the missing link in our quest for deeply satisfying wellness, is the only foundation that will make you want to nurture your precious body, mind and soul with regular feel-good-movement and beautifying whole foods. I know full well—the way you speak to yourself really does matter. Negativity spirals negativity. You cannot speak unkindly about your body and also make believe that you have a healthy, thriving relationship with it. It does not work.

Nothing good, productive or even remotely healthy can thrive in the toxic world of self-loathing and critical perfectionism. When you talk yourself down, you are only heaping self-manipulation, fear and shame on yourself. It shuts down any hope for positive change.

However, if you can reprogram your inner dialog, you will find the power to truly make your glowing healthy-licious new way of life. It is one thing to know this, and it's entirely another thing to turn it around. Changing your self-talk from unworthy to loving is the only way to bring your precious self to the place you long to be. Just for a brief moment, imagine how you would feel if your self-talk came to your heart as little love notes. Have you experienced the thrill of hope that surges into your soul when you feel safe in someone's abiding love and belief? It is incredibly empowering! In this place, even the world itself is not too big to conquer. There is nothing you cannot do inside of this perfect love. You are empowered with strength and focus, and you can do anything you set your mind to accomplish.

When your source of love and knowing comes from the wellspring of your own heart, your body becomes your home base. Trust me on this—loving your body for its wondrous gifts is truly the link to fully embracing a happy life. Transformation happens first in your heart and mind; your body will follow your loving lead. Nothing is more beautiful than the healthy-licious glow of a woman who has tuned in to the truth of her body and soul.

SIMPLE ACTION STEPS:

- Whenever a not-so-loving thought towards yourself pops into your mind, replace it with the thought "I am good enough."

- Whenever you doubt yourself, ask yourself whether you gave it your best, no matter the outcome. If the answer is "yes," you can be totally proud of yourself.

- Whenever perfectionism is taking over, very gently but sternly tell yourself that perfection does not exist. It is one way to make yourself feel bad, to procrastinate or to manipulate yourself into not so healthful ways of being.

- Whenever you feel down about your achievements or about yourself, think about all the things you are truly proud of in your life and how you made them happen. Honour this strength within you.

- Whenever you feel like you have made a mistake or let yourself down, embrace it as a learning curve which will help you to become even more awesome.

- There is nothing wrong with faking it until you make it. The fact is that most of us are much better at beating ourselves up than loving ourselves. It is a very odd thing, but we really are great at loving our daughters and sons, our partners, family, friends and pets—we are so kind and generous when it comes to others. However, when it comes to ourselves, we seem to struggle to offer the same love.

It is really important not to be too harsh with ourselves as we transition from self-loathing to self-compassion. It's important to remember that change doesn't come overnight. The longer we have been speaking unkindly to ourselves, the longer it will take us to recondition our brains and let go of this targeted negativity. Here is the bridge: Pretend you love yourself until you can truly and authentically do so. It's still better to say nice things to yourself, even if you cannot yet believe them, than not say them at all.

Eat like you love yourself. Move like you love yourself. Speak like you love yourself. Act like you love yourself. Just love yourself!!

THROUGH THE PAIN OF CHANGE

Let's be freaking honest; change is super hard and can be pretty scary. It means venturing out of your comfort zone and trying something new, plus it costs more energy and time than sticking with the old ways. This is because it means replacing old behaviours that no longer serve you with new ones. Those old ways are so deeply ingrained in your nervous system that you do them almost automatically. Overriding those habits with new ones takes you off autopilot and puts you in manual control. Until you develop a muscle memory (and a new neural pathway) for it, the changes will simply require more time and greater effort. If you are like me (and everyone else), you are terribly attached to your quirky ways and not entirely ready to give them up. The idea of transformation creates a prickly feeling of vulnerability because there is no guarantee the change will work in the way you envision it.

However, as awesome as that comfort zone is...it will not help you to reach your goals. Nor will it bring you to where you desire to be. If you keep doing what you have always done, even though it is cosy and easy and amazingly familiar, you will stay stuck in exactly that place. This means you are missing out on what could have been and who you could have become if you had only dared to try.

What if I told you that when it comes to change, we are all in the same boat? There is no easy way out and no quick fix. Most of us hesitate to bite the bullet and go the whole way to seeing things right through to the end. Unfortunately, though, sometimes we need a wake-up call or life lesson to get off our butts and make things happen (as was the case for me). My wish is for you to not let it come to that. Don't be harsh and neglect your gorgeous self as I did. I have made it my mission to empower you to embrace change as your first option so you never reach the breaking point that I did.

I do believe that talking openly about what it is you want to change and describing it exactly for what it is may help you change gears and accept that transformation is a process, not an event. This makes it less overwhelming by honouring the simple truth that we are human. Knowing we are not alone in our struggle gives comfort and keeps fresh power flowing.

Did you know that change comes in stages? I didn't, but I wish I had because I think it would have helped relieve my feelings of unworthiness and frustration when my attempts to change didn't work out straight away. If I had known this tango of to'ing and fro'ing—two steps forward and one step back—was part of the whole process, I would have felt far more empowered and accepting with the entire journey. Hopefully, by observing these stages of change, you can smile at yourself when you notice a back step and feel proud because it means that whatever you are doing *is* working...you are right in the middle of your difficult but beautiful process of leaving your old self behind and saying "Hi!" to the new, vibrant, radiant YOU that you are becoming.

CHANGE IS INDIVIDUAL

If you are anything like me, sometimes you feel insecure about yourself and your capabilities. It is important to acknowledge the fact that each person's transformation is individual. This is not so much because our bodies are made differently, but rather because there are so many right ways to change. When the pain of staying in your comfort zone hurts more than taking on the unfamiliar work of transformation, you are ready to make the leap of faith.

Truly, there is no such thing as *perfect timing*. When you come to believe that you deserve to feel strong and healthy and powerful—that you are a match for your dreams—you are ready. Believing that you are already enough liberates your mind, enabling you to focus and your soul to fully trust your intuition. Your whole gorgeous self will radiate with energy and vitality. You are so done being stuck in the old patterns of shame and frustration.

I invite you to get curious about what your process of change will look like. If you are a visual thinker like I am, you might envision it in the shape of a Valentine's heart. Perhaps making yourself a priority looks like a big fat tick on your life list. Or possibly your inner eye sees it as a scary-but-fun roller coaster ride that leaves you wobbly-kneed and thrilled at finding your strength. Are you becoming curious about that ride? Will it be gentle and slow or will it have sharp, quick turns that shake up your life in every good way that you have been secretly longing for? Fortunately, unlike a roller coaster, when it comes to your journey of transformation, you are in charge of the direction you take. This one is in your hands, and it is up to you to take it the way that is exactly right for you.

Each time I find myself approaching another opportunity to upgrade my life, I like to step back and imagine myself smiling at all those jittery insecurities. It reminds me that those silly doubts were just my mind playing tricks on me to keep me safe. Can you find a way to wink at yourself when things get tricky and just press forward in this direction? You are exactly where you need and want to be, with a wide, happy smile of *I-got-this* on your beautiful, courageous face.

CHANGE AND SELF-SABOTAGE

Let's get to the tricky bits. The whole psychological side of change reaches far back to our childhoods and the experiences that formed those beliefs we hold deeply within us about ourselves. In fact, these may be so deep that we might not even be aware of them.

Have you ever played with the idea that what is keeping you away from becoming the most vibrant, radiant version of yourself is fear? It may be fear of failure or, surprisingly, it may be fear of success. Maybe you hold excess weight as a physical protection against abuse and releasing it leaves you feeling vulnerable, bare and naked? Who would you be as a vibrant, healthy, strong woman? Would this throw you into a complete identity crisis? Would this require a reconciliation between your two ways of being? Are you utterly convinced within your deepest self that failure is inevitable? Do you shield yourself from the shame of failure by subconsciously sabotaging your efforts to become your healthy-licious best self?

Over the years, I have been so guilty of this. I struggle with a deep belief that I am unworthy. It has been really tricky not to create my world around these limiting beliefs, but I am not giving up on myself—not now, not ever. I would not be here on this earth if I had a "give up" mindset. (My mother would have aborted me if I had not been so good at hiding.) So, I will keep pushing away, as much as I can, that voice that lies to me from time to time.

I want you to do the same. You **are** worth living your best life. Whatever your story...you are not the story. You are not your limiting beliefs. You are a divine goddess—a gift to the world. Because of you, our world is a better place, so make sure you never give up on yourself. It is time to uncover the best that you are.

Whatever your reason for self-sabotage, be prepared for it to happen. We are complex human beings, and the more profound the hurt, the more difficulty we have in letting go of such seemingly protective layers of self-manipulation. Having said that, there is enormous power in becoming aware of such tendencies. The more willing you are to embrace yourself with all your difficult layers of previous experiences, the stronger you will be in quieting the ways in which those old ghosts try to haunt you.

WHEN YOU FALL OFF YOUR HEALTHY WAGON

Have you ever fallen off the wagon of your new commitment to health? Does that fall sink you with doubt and reinforce your old beliefs that you just don't have what it takes to thrive? You might start telling yourself a story that says, "Well. I've done it again. The damage is done, so I might as well just enjoy myself and not keep trying to change this." You might tell yourself that you are simply not able to do it or that you are not good enough or strong enough. The fall and the negative self-talk happen to the best of us. If we allow these old ideas to have too much power over us, we are truly moving away from a healthy place.

I want you to try something new. Instead of throwing in the towel and giving up, I invite you to simply acknowledge that you have fallen off. Smile big at yourself and jump right back on. No need for guilt or beating yourself up for it. No damage done. All that happened is that you fell off for whatever reason and now you are back on. You have not turned into a bad person because of it. And no, you have not ruined all your best efforts just because of this one slip-up. Remember that your healthy journey can look like a little tango dance, and that is okay.

It's not the piece of cake you ate or the fact that you skipped your exercise routine that shakes your confidence. Nope. Nor is it what you did or did not do. It is what you hold as your mindset that determines what you do next. Your mindset either reminds you that you are determined to do whatever it takes to look and feel amazing or else it triggers a downward, negative, fatalistic spiral. Please don't let a negative mindset derail you on this journey.

Instead, look into the mirror and gift yourself with a big smile, dust yourself off and go right back to what makes you feel beautiful, worthy and amazing...which is jumping right back into the healthy-licious YOU. Best news of all—there is absolutely no limit to how often you can jump back onto this wagon that brings the best out in you. In fact, the more often you jump back on, the more graceful become your leaps. True fact. So, if you are serious about your desire to glow with health and beauty from the inside out, the key is to focus on how quickly you can get back into the saddle. The fall does not matter at all.

WEIGHT-LOSS

It pains me to see that most weight-loss journeys begin from a place of hate, or loathing, or shame towards our own bodies. It almost feels like we are angry with our bodies for not being the shape or size we want or expect them to be. I'm here to say, "It is not our bodies' faults."

The truth is, at any given moment, your body is busy trying to do its utmost best for you. Is this not enough reason to love your body and to be grateful to it for being there for you no matter what? No matter how much you loathe it, or how unhappy you are with the way it looks, no matter how much you offend or punish it, it just continues to be good to you. Your body always has your back!

Sometimes, however, this backup doesn't work out in your favour. This is where you fall out of tune with what your physical self truly needs. For example, when you confuse the signs of fatigue for emotional hunger, you might eat more food instead of getting more rest. It happens when you forget how to directly identify your body's cues and act accordingly. It has nothing to do with your body being wrong or unkind, and it has nothing to do with you being wrong or weak-willed.

I know from my own experience how very destructive to my physical self this out-of-tune approach can be. I observe this daily among girls and women of all ages. I witness them beating themselves up for not being in their "perfect" bodies and it creates more pain, more drama and more resistance. It widens the gap between where they are and where they want to be.

It strikes me as incredibly sad that we are trying to go on a journey of body transformation, hating the body that will not only take us on the journey, but is the very thing we want to transform. We expect it to do something great as we bombard it with negativity. Step back and observe this from a distance. This cannot work. Do you think you would have much success changing your kids, your partner or your best friend by shouting at them? Will hateful stares, nasty comments and tight-fisted punches to their vulnerable backs inspire them to greatness? I very much doubt it.

Well, guess what? The same is true for you. So, let's begin this whole journey with love. At the risk of repeating myself, this is the only way sustainable change is possible. After all, every long-lasting, happy relationship needs love as its solid foundation, right? I am not talking about the shallow, ego-driven pride that feels superior to everyone else; I mean your heart that loves all of your body as beautiful and worthy and acceptable. This heart loves you with a kindness and a blindness. It sees the whole of you, accepts all of you, and honours every part of you for performing its best functions all day, every day.

Can you love the softness of your belly for having been so magical as to allow you to give birth to your child instead of hating your stretch marks? Can you embrace your thighs as strong even if you think they should be skinny? Can you welcome butts or upper arms that wobble and be proud of all that they have lived through? Can you somewhere in your heart find for yourself the same kind of love and acceptance you have for your best friend despite her not looking like a perfect supermodel? Do you think you can do this? Or at least try? If so, you are ready to start a successful weight-loss journey.

I want to share the story of my very dear friend who lives across the oceans in America. She is beautiful and stunning, inside and out. She has this amazing glow of total goddess to her. She is one of the strongest people I know. She is also super brave. My dear, beautiful friend recently stepped away from years of domestic violence in its most brutal form. She decided to change, knowing that the old life she was living did not serve her anymore, and she understood that she could not be or give to the world the way she was meant to. Staying in such a toxic relationship meant saying "no" to her greatness. It meant being toxic to herself. I would lie if I said her journey of walking away from hate and embracing love has been easy, but with every step that she takes, her life gets more colourful, more magical and more worth it. She is gaining the courage to own more of her dazzling beauty and awesomeness. However, she is still stuck in an overweight body she cannot love just yet...a body which protected her from more violence—a body that helped her survive. She relied on sugar to bring sweetness and comfort into a too-painful life. Her body shape or size does not make her any less magic, but it hinders her from living her best life. Her knees hurt and her body is exhausted.

I want you to know that whatever your story, whatever your reason for holding on to more weight than that which makes you feel good, you are not your past. You are not your body weight or the number on the scale. You are the unique and beautiful YOU and are worth loving yourself for it. You are worth living your best life in a body that feels light, happy, strong and vibrant. You can at any given moment in time decide to leave your own old story to change, to turn your back to the old and start anew. When you do, do it with love!

Sleep

Sleep truly affects all aspects of our lives. If you have ever been sleep-deprived, you know what I am talking about. (I'm sure every woman with children agrees—this is the toughest bit about being a mum.) Not being able to replenish your tired brain and body overnight with deep, restful, feel-good sleep is the worst torture of all. It changes the way all our body systems function and it can get pretty scary. In my case, this is the difference between being a zombie and a radiant, I-can-do-this-and-I-will action doll. I wish I was joking, but I am not. Ever since my head operation I have been a horrible sleeper, struggling to fall asleep and stay asleep, waking at the slightest noise. To get a deep, restorative, full night's sleep is something I have missed for so many years. I thought it was just a consequence of my surgery that I had to accept, but the more I practise Nutrition and Health Coaching, the more I have learned that poor sleep is common among women. This has given me a desire to heal my sleep patterns and to empower others to heal theirs, too.

The effects of sleep deprivation on your nervous system:

- Reduced memory function.
- Reduced concentration, focus, and clarity.
- Increased feelings of anxiety, nervousness, and depression.
- Reduced ability to cope with the stress of life and difficult situations.
- Increased irritability and moodiness.

The effects of sleep deprivation on your endocrine system:

- Increased production of ghrelin (feel-hungry hormone).
- Reduced production of leptin (feel-full hormone).
- Increased production of stress hormones (lowers immunity, increases risk of systemic inflammation).
- Increased levels of insulin (linked to increased storage of body fat, especially around your middle. Arggh!!)

The effects of sleep deprivation on your immune system:

- Reduced immunity.
- Increased risk of systemic inflammation (linked to increased risk of cardiovascular disease).

The effects of sleep deprivation on your cardiovascular system:

- Increased risk of cardiovascular disease, especially stroke and heart attack, due to lowered ability to keep our blood vessels and heart strong and healthy; inflammation increases blood pressure and blood glucose, which leads to increased calcium deposits in our arteries.
- Elevated triglyceride levels (linked to heart disease).
- Decreased "good' cholesterol.

The effects of sleep deprivation on your digestive system:

- Increased hunger.
- Reduced satiety.
- Reduced digestion and proper absorption of nutrients.
- Increased stomach upset, indigestion, and heartburn.

The effects of sleep deprivation on your respiratory system

- Increased risk of respiratory infections due to compromised immunity.
- Increased risk of common colds and flu.

I don't know about you, but as far as I'm concerned, this is a pretty convincing list. I can only speak for myself, but when I have not slept well, I am not my usual self. Everything seems so much harder and I feel far less capable of dealing with my life. I cannot find the right words, I seem to forget what I had just been talking about, my patience for dealing with stress is nearly gone, my body seems to move with less flow, bounce, and buoyancy, and the whole world seems to run in super slow, everything-is-an-effort motion. I absolutely hate being in such a dull, day-dazing state...it seems such a waste of my precious time.

In recent times, transforming my own sleepless life has become an urgent call to me, knowing that if I can change my sleep, then I can also help you change yours. I have made it my mission to experiment with a wide variety of holistic strategies to improve the quality of my sleep and sleep patterns. To say that I have become VERY protective of my sleep is a grand understatement, sometimes to the chagrin of my family. While I am generous in many areas of my life, I am not necessarily so serving when it comes to my sleep. Sorry, princess daughters, there will be no up-till-all-hours sleepovers at our house. You might laugh at the measures I take to ensure a good night's sleep (and world peace!), but they work, and that's all that matters to me. I do not want to spend my life dragging my backside around in a zombie-like stupor.

TRANSFORM YOUR LIVING-DEAD ZOMBIE INTO A RESTED SLEEPING BEAUTY

Getting seven to eight hours of good quality sleep each night is vital to your health. While some women may find they can truly get by with less, it's best to tune into your body to find the truth about how much sleep your body requires.

It is so tempting to prolong your evenings by going to bed later so that you can fit more into the day. Busy days and meeting all the demands of your family leave little time for self-nurture and self-care. For me, finding myself in a finally-quiet home often means staying awake simply to soak in the beauty of the silence. Let's be honest, though, you're already so overtired that those quiet evening hours are more likely filled with less-than-nurturing activities like watching TV, catching up on some reading or scrolling through social media.

Stepping into your sleeping power and making this sleep-boosting switch will not only allow you to fully use your awake time to your best abilities, but is also very likely to add some real quality time into those shorter, but more enjoyable evenings of yours.

I challenge you to commit to going to bed 1 hour earlier than you usually do for 1 month to make a habit of this positive change.

SUPPORT YOUR HEALTHY-LICIOUS SLEEP ACTION STEPS:

- *Establish a mind-calming, body-relaxing evening routine*
    - It's important to signal your body that it's time to step away from the non-stop action of the day. This happens in an evening routine—a sequence of self-nurturing actions that you are willing to perform every evening at approximately the same time. This could be using calming essential oils, reading a book for pleasure, listening to calming music, or soaking in a warm bath or taking a relaxing shower. In no time at all, your body will come to recognise and relish these "it's almost time to sleep" signals and support your efforts. The more punctual you are with your new sleeping pattern of self-love, the more quickly you will reset your circadian (day/night) rhythms, you will heal your sleep cycle and soon be rewarded with deeply rejuvenated REM (Rapid Eye Movement) sleep.

- **Wind down without electronics**
    - Our dependence upon our devices has come at a high price to our sleep. The blue light emitted from our screens horribly disrupts our circadian rhythms. Instead of inviting our tired bodies and minds to shut down, they promote wakefulness. I promise I'm not suggesting that you are not to watch TV or write those important business emails in the evening. Rather, I am inviting you to set aside some time apart from those things before you set your head on your pillow for the night. Your body and mind need a very literal separation from your time spent on electronic devices to register that it is time to switch off and adjust to that change.

- *Create your perfect sleep haven*
    - For your sleep to be deeply restorative, it is essential to create a calm environment that invites sleepiness. Shut out anything that could possibly disrupt your rest. Keep electronics and any work-related materials out of your bedroom. Your bedroom should be a place of physical rejuvenation, a sanctuary, a haven—it is for sleep and for sex. It is not a place for anything that requires much mental effort.
    - It is best to shut out all the light that you possibly can, keeping your space very dark, quiet, and cool. (My inner sleep nerd requires my eye mask, ear plugs, and the investment of expensive pillows so I can drift off to Planet Dream without my neck feeling stiff the next day.)

- **If you choose to drink alcohol, drink moderately and pair it with dinner and stay hydrated with water**
    - It is true that a glass of red wine in the evening can help you fall asleep more quickly. Unfortunately, it is also true that alcohol interferes with your biorhythm, or your internal biological clock, which regulates most of your body's processes, including metabolism, immunity, cognition, mood, sleep, energy, and more. As a result, you will be tossing and turning around in bed rather than falling into a deep rejuvenating sleep, leaving your fatigued self without time to make the slightest attempt at any form of recovery.
    - Not only that, alcohol blocks the REM sleep cycle where dreaming occurs and the body is energized. Your brain secretes the neurotransmitter acetylcholine during REM sleep,

which processes memories and provides energy to your mind and body. Skipping REM sleep will leave you feeling, when you wake up, as though you did not really sleep at all, with a brain fog so thick that even sugar and caffeine don't really help to clear it.

- *Nurture your body with easily-digested food*
  - o In our hectic lives, we rarely give attention to refuelling our bodies with wholesome foods. More often than not, we hurry through a skimpy lunch and forget altogether about morning and afternoon snacks, arriving home to dinner in the evening starved for food. We are so incredibly hungry and have not given any time in the day to nurturing ourselves with good food, leaving us now in danger of over-eating. This overload of food taxes the stomach, requiring it to labour in the evening, rather than rest. If you are serious about sleeping well at night, I invite you to attend to your body through the day, being mindful of eating more while you are active, and more often to avoid blood sugar highs and lows. Leaving the harder-to-digest foods (fatty foods or red meat) for your active time and your lighter, easily digestible foods for the evening prepares your body to move more naturally to your resting phase at the end of the day.

- *Quit troublesome foods*
  - o Are there foods in your diet that cause you immediate regret when you eat them? Foods that make you look almost instantly five months pregnant? Foods that make you tired, cause gas or make you feel uncomfortable and uneasy? Stop eating those things! Your body is signalling you through those unpleasant feelings that it does not favour those particular foods. Those foods are not made for your unique body and your digestive system struggles to metabolize them. The most common culprits of this digestive incompatibility are extreme spices, gluten, artificial colours, added sugar, and highly-processed foods. Consuming these toxic-for-you foods at night puts your digestion and your immunity on high alert, denying them the rest your body deserves when it's time to sleep.

- *Enjoy food and drinks that boost your sleep quality*
  - o Would you be surprised to know that many whole foods naturally contain nutrients that support healthy sleep? Almonds are one of my favourite sleep-promoting foods. Almonds contain melatonin, a sleep regulating hormone and they are a rich source of magnesium, which helps decrease inflammation and improve sleep quality.
  - o Try adding these sleep-great-foods to your arsenal — walnuts, kiwifruit, oatmeal, bananas, dark chocolate, passionflower tea, warm hot chocolate with raw cacao, turkey, and fish high in omega 3 fatty acids. Remember however, that simply because these foods have amazing sleep-promoting properties, they do not come with a free pass for over-indulgence. Even if you eat all the right foods, if you eat too much too late, you will counteract the whole point. You will not only not sleep better, you will also gain unwanted weight and all that comes with it.

Let me restate this: there is truly no more effective way to boost your energy, health, memory, beauty and youth than by enjoying your regular 7-8 hours of deep, good quality sleep. It is during such restorative sleep that your body releases the many toxins accumulated during your busy day, that it secretes youthful growth hormones, and it's when your body processes memory and creates room for new learning. It is true for everyone. When sleep quality is poor, our mental and physical performance is greatly reduced, our hormones become all jumbled up, our bellies grow fat, and we feel and look many years older than we actually are.

It is high time that we all make good quality sleep a priority in our overworked and overstressed lives. Too many of us are stuck in a sleepless cycle of wired exhaustion. It is time to step out of such destructive patterns. I have been there. I hear and feel you, I truly do. There is nothing worse than not being able to recover properly during the night to then equip us with sufficient new vitality to manage our crazily busy days.

You do not have to sacrifice all of your evening pleasures and social events for sleep, but it is essential that you know what your balanced life looks like. Sleep is sacred and an incredibly important piece in the puzzle of your best, most vital, radiant self. Look, if I can end the sleepless overdrive of my own life, leading to more ignited and productive daytime activity, you can do it, too. It is far easier and more straightforward than you think it is.

Stress Less

I know, it is easier said than done, but we have to wake up and get serious about doing something to change our stress levels. This health threat is literally killing us.

CORTISOL AND HOW IT AFFECTS YOUR BODY

As we know, our amazing body always has our back...always. When the body is exposed to stress, it responds in an instant with adrenaline rising and sugar being dumped into the bloodstream. At the same time, cortisol and growth hormone levels rise, too. You are ready to fight that tiger, flee from his presence, or freeze, depending on the circumstance. It is all about survival. In the olden days, when the threat was over, the body returned to its normal state. But in today's world, the threat never fully goes away which means the body never gets to return to stasis. Chronic stress then exceeds our ability to cope with and respond well to our everyday challenges.

Chronically high cortisol levels really mess with our overall health and well-being. They result in:

- Blood sugar imbalances.
- Increased fat around the middle (which has been linked to a greater risk of heart disease, cancer, diabetes, obesity, and higher levels of cholesterol).
- Higher blood pressure.
- Lower bone density and increased risk of osteoporosis.
- Thinning skin and slower capacity to heal wounds.
- Higher levels of inflammation in the body.
- Lowered immunity.
- Increased risk of thyroid issues.
- Decreased cognitive functioning and significant memory loss.
- Increased risk of depression.
- Increased risk of insomnia.
- Increased risk of dementia.
- Increased risk of Cushing disease.
- Increased indigestion and gastric upsets.
- Increased risk of adrenal tumour.
- Lowered fertility.

HOW CAN YOU EFFECTIVELY MANAGE STRESS?

At the very least, nurture your precious body with wholesome foods and move regularly with feel-good exercise. Do not underestimate the power of this solid foundation in addressing your skyrocketing cortisol levels. This is the beginning, but it may not be enough. Depending on your personal situation and genetic make-up, you may want to become far more specific in addressing whatever is throwing your stress levels overboard.

What else can you do to manage your stress better and improve your entire wellbeing?

Have you heard about the four A's of stress management? I love their simplicity and effectiveness. I hope you do, too. These principles are great reminders of how intuitive we really are—we know these things deep inside us. Somehow, we forget how to apply what we know and we allow ourselves to ignore our inner wisdom.

WANT TO STRESS LESS? HERE ARE YOUR HOT LEADS!

- **Avoid unnecessary stress**
  - Learn to say "no" to people and things that do not align with your situation. I know how hard this is! It feels like you are mistreating someone or rejecting them or being unkind. But let's be honest, we are no good to anyone if we have run ourselves into the ground.
  - Get clear on which people or situations add stress to your life. Choose your priorities wisely and lovingly safeguard them. Do not accept more demands on your time and spirit that you are not willing to give. If this means choosing not to answer a friend's call to chat, but instead waiting until you are able to be wholeheartedly with him/her, you are practicing self-love and healthy stress management. Your friend will love you all the more for it.

- **Alter the situation**
  - These questions can give you some alternatives to deal with the demands that come your way.
    - ❷ How can I change this knocks-me-on-my-butt situation into a I-can-do-this opportunity?
    - ❷ How can I use my time more efficiently?
    - ❷ Am I communicating openly and effectively? Do I need to change the way I am communicating?
    - ❷ Are my ideals of perfection making my life harder?
    - ❷ Can I be more flexible in the situation?
    - ❷ Am I complicating something that can be simple?
    - ❷ Can I modify my approach to be softer?

- **Adapt your stressor**
  - This is my favourite stress-less technique because *it just works*. It instantly transforms a supercharged situation into humble bliss. Try it for yourself!
    - ‣ Reframe the stressful situation. Instead of seeing a disruptive event as a threat, try calling it an empowering learning curve. See the signs of life being about to change for the better.
    - ‣ Look at the bigger picture. What is the opportunity that is opening now?

- ▸ Trade negative self-talk with positive, self-nurturing, loving words. You have not failed at anything! You are a work in progress—that is the truth for each of us.

- ▸ Evaluate and manage your expectations. Is your goal real? Is it possible? Is it manageable? Or have you set your expectations titanically high, exponentially adding to your stress? How can you frame your goal into bite-size steps?

- ▸ Pause and be thankful for all that you have. Trade your gripes for gratitude.

- **Accept the things you cannot change**
  - o I have spent a long time in my life chasing ideas in my mind instead of accepting things or situations for what they are. This is neither constructive nor helpful. Even if you are the most determined, most powerful force of nature known to the world, there are some circumstances that simply are what they are and that is okay. Choosing acceptance over resistance is so liberating!

  - o It is far better for our fatigued adrenal glands when we identify those things which simply are *what they are*. Then we can choose our healthy responses to those challenges as self-caring strategies. Instead of bracing myself against those unchangeable things, I now embrace those situations as beautiful opportunities to practise acceptance—I know that I am exactly where I'm meant to be.

  - o Want to know how to begin this transformation? Just take baby steps. Share with someone you love and trust what torments you. Get out of your head and put it out there where you can see it for what it is, then you can decide how you will respond to it in the future.

MORE HANDS-ON ANTI-STRESS ACTION STEPS

- **Practise Mindfulness**
  - o Have the constant demands of your life twisted you into a cortisol-ridden, anxious bombshell? Has a mind racing with a thousand thoughts become your new, unhappy normal? If I have described you, then it is high time to introduce mindfulness to your gloomy, overstretched, non-stop psyche. Can you remember the last time you paused to drink in the sweetness of flowers in full bloom or absorbed your thoughtful gaze with the azure blueness of the ocean? Do you remember the happy, chirpy song of springtime?

  - o If it has been far too long, let me invite you to change this. Return to the wonder of becoming a vivid observer of the magic that surrounds you. I know, I can hear you saying, "If only it was that easy." Being mindful, like anything worthwhile, takes practise. It cannot somehow mysteriously vanish your worries (shame that!), but learning to engage mindfully in your world becomes a warm hug to your tormented mind. The more often you do this, the more natural to you this way of comforting perception will become.

  - o Mindfulness lives everywhere—so the next time you shower, try focusing your attention on the sensations the water brings you. Notice how those warm little life-giving water droplets feel on your beautiful skin. Such simple pleasures are the difference between happiness and misery.

- *Write a daily gratitude journal*
  - o The thought of adding another chore into your life could make you cringe with doubt. How on earth can you possibly fit one more thing into your day? That was my reaction, too. However, happily looking through a 5-minute-gratitude window and counting your blessings has incredible mood-lifting power. Trade it up for the monotony of TV or social media. Write down 5 things that you are truly grateful for. It is quickly done and is so much more uplifting than the energy spent following the world's tragedies on the news. Of course, how you spend your time is a deeply personal decision. For me, I have discovered that prioritizing my mental health is a no-cost decision that blends easily into my day. It makes all the difference for me in mastering my life in a happy, efficient way. It has replaced the mind-numbing, heavy, fearful, not-coping-well behaviours I used to have. Looking back, I feel almost silly and ashamed of my previous self for arguing against such an empowering practise. It takes so little time and the return on my investment is huge. Now, it is gratitude lists every day for me. When will you start writing yours?

- **Rest and re-balance**
  - o As far as I am concerned, everything is far worse when I'm tired. Fatigue feeds my worries, aggravates my fears, and makes me less capable of coping with everything that life throws at me. My stress levels spiral out of control. I have to say, it's not very attractive. Please do not make the mistake of confusing success with allowing stress to rule your life!

  - o I encourage you, in addition to practising your revitalising sleep habits, to find little pockets of deep, stress-free calm during your day. Creating the space to nurture your precious mind, body and soul throughout each day is vital to your entire well-being. Of course, these bits of revitalizing, peaceful serenity that fit into new little windows of time will look different from one person to the next, so let me share what mine looks like and what works for me. Maybe you will find a gem that works for you, too. My favourite (most time-effective) ones are:
    - Listening to a transformative, empowering, feel-good podcast whenever I am cooking, ironing, or just driving around.
    - Looking at or listening to something that makes me laugh...really laugh...so hard that my eyes start watering and my belly hurts.
    - Belly breathing. How it looks: I put one hand on my belly and inflate my midsection so my hand moves away (the more you can blow up/out your belly, the better) and then fully deflate my midsection, so my hand moves back towards me. I like to take 3-5 breaths like this, whenever I feel my stress levels surging high in acute situations (such as those crazy working mum situations where my princess girls are fighting in a not very princess-like way, while my mobile phone is sending continuous work-related messages through, just as I'm trying to get dinner on the table). Whilst belly-breathing, I like to visualise that I am inhaling gloriously, refreshing calmness and exhaling all of the stress, worries and negativity, letting it all go with the flow of my out breath.
    - Cuddling my cute cat, Charlie. I stop whatever I'm doing and pay him some devoted attention while he lovingly obliges by calming my stressed mind. There is nothing more soothing to me than listening to his purring and feeling his beautiful fur rubbing against

my skin. To him, happiness is that simple...and magically some of his simple happiness always transfers to me.

- Turning on a diffuser to infuse the fragrance of some relaxing, calming or revitalising essential oil (or a mix of several). Alternatively, I might apply a few drops to my wrists or my temples or rub them gently into the soles of my feet.

- Lying down with my back flat on the ground and with my legs up against the wall in a 90-degree angle for a few minutes. Try it! Notice how your legs will start to tingle all over as your blood flow is reversed. This might feel very unusual to you at first. For me, it is one of the quickest and most effective ways to recharge my body.

- Taking a 20-minute power nap.

- Revitalising my body with this little nurturing flow technique I developed. I start by going into a deep, standing forward fold. I then roll my spine up to standing, while pressing my hands onto my shins and legs as I go, activating all those nerves and meridians in my legs. Upon standing, I like to bring my arms overhead and then dive with a flat back and straight arms forward as much and for as long as I can before rounding down again into a deep forward fold. Repeat for 6-8 rounds.

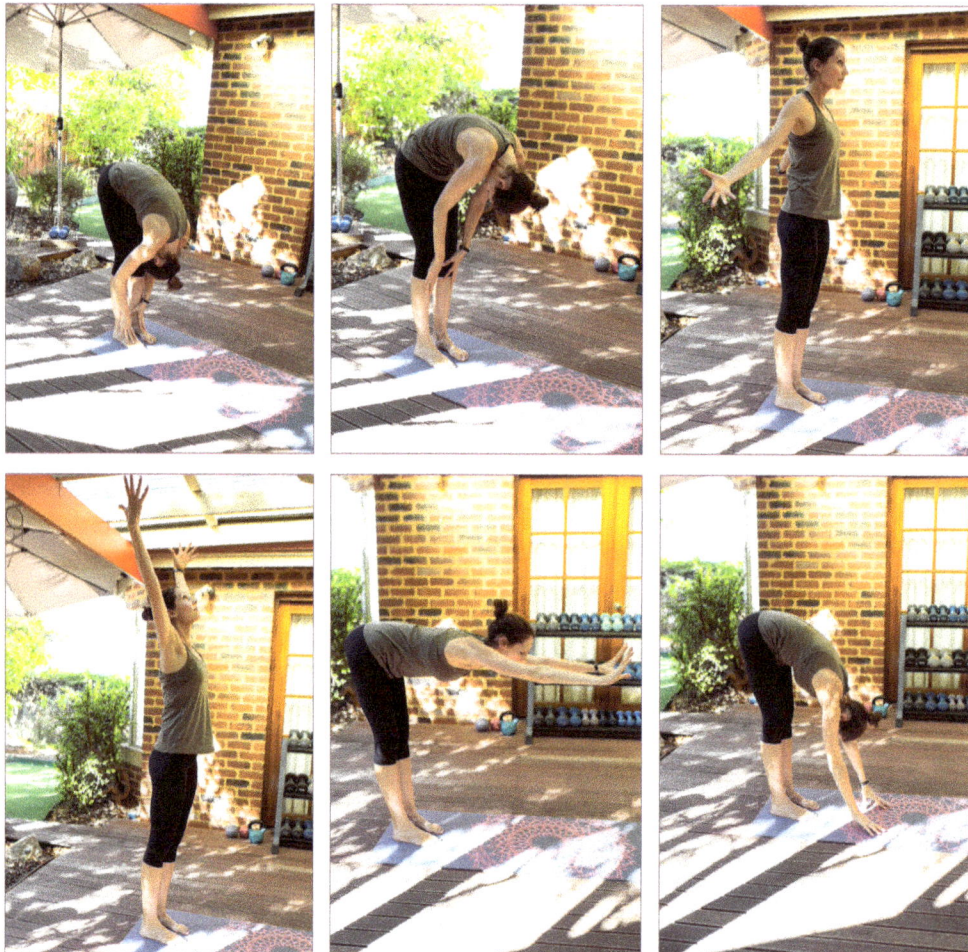

- Doing 3-4 slow sun salutations.
- Sitting for five or more minutes outside in the garden or on the veranda, listening to all the sounds that nature offers, while feeling the sun kissing my face.
- Sitting down with a cup of warm, soothing herbal tea (chocolate-chili has to be my all-time favourite!)
- Listening to a positive mantra or piece of music that makes me feel good, cheerful and happy.

MANAGING STRESS THROUGH YOUR FOOD CHOICES

Consider avoiding foods that add more stress to your body

In times of high stress, our bodies have to dig deep to maintain health and well-being. The greater the intensity, and the more prolonged the state of stress is, the more overtime our bodies are putting in. It seems only fair to try and support the body's strenuous endeavours here by not adding more fuel to the stress fire. There are particular foods that add more stress to our poor system. I invite you to give yourself a break from them while you are trying to rebound to a state of more balanced vitality.

Foods that spike our stress levels are:

- All foods high in refined sugar.
- All foods high in salt.
- Foods containing gluten.
- Foods containing unhealthy fats (especially trans-fatty acids).
- Alcohol.
- Coffee (I am not saying coffee in itself is a bad thing and needs to be avoided, but when your stress levels are off the chart, so to speak, it is definitely not the drink that will assist your inner glow, calm and vitality.)
- Any foods that contain artificial colours, fillers, or preservatives.
- All highly processed foods and pre-cooked foods (unless pre-cooked by you, of course).

Consider replacing these with plenty of healthy-licious foods that soothe your brain chemistry. And yes, it is possible to eat your way to greater balance.

MY TOP 6 RECOMMENDED FOODS FOR BRINGING MORE CALMNESS TO YOUR HECTIC LIFE:

1. Foods that are high in folate

Amongst the most stress relieving foods are those that are high in folate. Folate is needed to make certain neurotransmitters such as serotonin and dopamine. Therefore, eating more of this vitamin can prevent deficiencies and help your body to produce more of those feel-good hormones.

Foods that are particularly rich in folate include dark leafy green vegetables, asparagus, avocados, brussels sprouts, broccoli, and citrus fruits.

2. Foods that are a rich source of magnesium

Magnesium is able to regulate your nervous system and reduce your stress in more than just one way. This amazing mineral is a precursor for the neurotransmitters serotonin. This means that a diet high in magnesium will help to better regulate our emotions and boost our general well-being. In addition, magnesium supports our adrenal glands, which become more depleted the more stressed we are. By consuming more of this anti-stress mineral, we can replenish our stores of magnesium and thus prevent our cells from being over-reactive.

Foods that are fantastic sources of magnesium include raw cacao powder, pumpkin seeds, seaweed, beans, leafy green vegetables, avocados, brown rice, and bananas.

3. Foods that hold high levels of vitamin C

Vitamin C is the anti-stress vitamin in that it is quickly able to counteract the release of cortisol and helps to clear the stress hormone out of our bloodstream. It thus prevents cortisol levels from staying elevated as well as prevents high spikes of blood glucose which are part of our normal response to stressful situations.

Foods that are particularly high in vitamin C are berries, red and green capsicum, kiwi fruits, kale, parsley, cilantro, leafy green vegetables, broccoli, brussels sprouts, and oranges.

4. Foods that comprise large amounts of the essential amino acid, tryptophan

Tryptophan is an essential amino acid which the body cannot produce on its own and therefore has to obtain it from food sources. One of the many functions of tryptophan is its ability to convert to serotonin which is associated with mood regulation. High levels of serotonin in the brain can reduce feelings of stress and instead promote feelings of relaxation and contentedness.

Foods that contain considerable amounts of tryptophan include organic turkey, chicken, pumpkin seeds, dairy, bananas, raw cacao powder, rolled oats, tofu, eggs, and salmon.

5. Foods rich in omega-3 fatty acids

In our modern western diets, we often tend to eat an unhealthy balance of omega-6 fatty acids in preference to the healthy omega-3 fatty acids. Omega-3 fatty acids are essential to our well-being, in particular to the health of our brains and nervous systems. Not consuming enough of these brain-nourishing omega-3 fatty acids can lead to inflammation in the brain and disruption of cell communication which then is linked to further stress, anxiety and depression.

Foods that are fantastic sources of omega-3 fatty acids include wild caught salmon, flaxseeds, and walnuts.

6. Fermented foods

Fermented foods contain beneficial gut micro-organisms which fight off harmful bacteria, and thus help to maintain a balance between good and bad bacteria in the digestive system. There is increasing research that suggests there is a direct link between the microbiome in the gut and the state of our mind and nervous system. The healthier and more balanced our intestinal micro-organisms, the better we are able to produce the neurotransmitter, serotonin. This then means we are much more capable to deal with our life's stressors in a positive and effective way.

Great examples of fermented foods are yoghurt, kefir, sauerkraut, sourdough bread, miso, kimchi and kombucha.

I know I'm a bit of a healthy food nerd, but isn't it empowering to know that you can cook up a stress-busting storm to help you stay more on top of everything that life throws at you? It really can be that easy to find your healthy food happy place.

NOURISHING YOURSELF THE ANTI-INFLAMMATORY WAY—IT WORKS!

I acknowledge that nurturing your precious mind, body and soul with wholesome brain-boosting and rebalancing foods might still not be enough to bounce back to your most vibrant, radiant, feel-good self. In fact, I have experienced in my own body how prolonged stress without adequate coping mechanisms can foster inflammation and how such inflammation then attacks those parts of my body that are genetically weaker. I have, among other things, a long line of severe arthritis in my family history and it rears its ugly head when my body is stressed and inflamed. I'm sure you would agree, it's not a great look for a personal trainer to be crawling out of bed stiff with arthritic joints. I may be many things, but I have always been determined to never, ever give up. I have already experienced once how powerful the self-healing mechanisms of our bodies truly are, so when I have felt this arthritic condition coming on, I've tapped into that same power again. I started by actively addressing my stressors from the outside with better coping mechanisms, such as more rest and more self-nurturing. At the same time, I began the process of researching all the foods that foster inflammation and those that do not.

I had soon committed to healing ways of self-care with lots of little baby steps to the best of my ability and with what little time I had available. I committed to nourishing my body only with foods that I believe to be anti-inflammatory. It was not easy for me to give up on certain foods at first. I have to confess that I had a secret love affair with yoghurt, of all things. Yep...yoghurt! Yoghurt is super healthy, but unfortunately, not for me. In hindsight, I do realise that it was more than a little romance. I can see now how I was craving yoghurt in a way you long for someone in an unhealthy relationship. You know this person is not doing you any good, but you are clinging onto him or her with fierceness. Like, it is the only person you could ever love or the only food that would nourish you in that way. The good thing is...I made a promise to myself and I was going to stand by that promise. So, I replaced my beloved Greek Dairy Yoghurt with almond milk and other plant substitutes. I made sure I fed my inflamed body with more omega-3 fatty acids. I stayed strict with not turning to any foods that could feed the inflammation. I was determined to extinguish and clear from my body the inflammation that was attacking it...and it worked! I have got my arthritis under control, no longer debilitating me, allowing me instead to jump out of bed like I used to. I want you to know that you, too, can impact on your genes and control the direction that life can take you.

Do you need an anti-inflammatory diet? If so, then this list is for you. It's time to renew and rebalance your beautiful body.

Avoid these:
- Trans-fatty acids such as those found in margarine, many baked goods like crackers, pastries and biscuits.
- All forms of refined sugar (once you feel better you can limit to 1-2 teaspoons of rice malt syrup per day).
- Dairy.
- Red meat and any processed meats.
- Refined grains (white flour, pasta, rice, etc)

- Coffee
- Alcohol (I would omit alcohol fully when you are starting off and once you feel better, you can enjoy 1 glass of good quality red bio wine 3 times per week, if you would like.)
- Grains that contain gluten.

Limit these:
- Omega-6 fatty acids (instead, introduce to your diet more omega-3 fatty acids to re-establish your body's natural balance) such as the following vegetable oils: sunflower, corn, soybean, and cottonseed oil.

- Saturated fats (they should stay under 10% of your total daily calorie intake) such as meat, butter, cheese, pastries, cakes, biscuits, and pies

- Dried fruits

- Black tea (limit to 2 per day)

- Dark store-bought chocolate (not lower than 75% of cocoa), make your own instead!!!

Enjoy these:
- Lots of vegetables and fruits in all the colours of the rainbow (at least 5-9 servings each day) in particular: dark berries; dark leafy green vegetables; dark grapes; cherries; cruciferous vegetables such as broccoli, cauliflower, brussels sprouts, and mustard greens; red cabbage; allium vegetables such as onions, spring onions, garlic, and leek; avocado.

- Lots of anti-inflammatory spices and herbs like turmeric, ginger, cinnamon, cloves, rosemary, sage, and thyme.

- Foods rich in omega-3 fatty acids such as walnuts, flaxseeds, chia seeds and linseeds and/or such oils, oily fish such as salmon, and sardines.

- Extra Virgin Olive oil, and olives.

- Whole-grains that are gluten free.

- Fish (at least twice per week).

- Plant protein such as lentils, tofu, and beans.

- White meat such as chicken and turkey.

- Lots of herbal infusions, filtered water, vegetable juices, fruit and vegetable smoothies, and green tea.

Obviously, adapting your diet in such a way can feel more restrictive. Therefore, I would like to invite you to stay open to listening to your own body, mind and soul at all times. Remember that nurturing your precious body is a fluid concept that only works by staying flexible and being able to adapt your diet (constantly) to your individual needs and changing circumstances. Also, remember to embrace these diet changes more as trading one thing with another, rather than simply omitting it. This is so important for you to be able to feel nurtured by your way of eating. Make it fun and make it work for you! Yes, you really can enjoy delicious meals and rid your body of inflammation at the same time. It feels and looks amazing!!!!

Just Breathe!

There is no denying that our crazy-busy, more-fast-paced-than-ever lives make us, collectively, super-stressed. "Stressed out of our minds," some would say. Our precious bodies carry the heavy symptoms of being so overstretched. As the cortisol builds up in our bodies, our waistlines grow, our cravings increase, and our overall well-being declines. Yet, we are too busy to sit down and breathe. To really breathe, without a cup of coffee, smart phone, or other electronic distraction at hand. I'm referring to being able to breathe in a way where we can let go of all the accumulated worry, anxiety, and pressure and forget about our endless to-do-lists...to be in a space where we allow our nervous systems to find balance and our hormones to readjust.

FIND YOUR MOST INTUITIVE, CALM, AND INSPIRED SELF THROUGH MEDITATION

When I first started to sit down and make time to breathe, I felt almost sick. My thoughts raced constantly through my overly worked mind. As I tried to stop those thoughts from going around and around in my head, I couldn't shake off a sense of "What on earth am I doing here? Am I wasting my precious time, sitting here on the ground, trying to quiet a mind that seems impossible to shut up?"

At times I felt I had my inner devil sitting on one shoulder and my angel Ruth on the other. The shoulder devil constantly shouted at me: "Go on, get up...continue on with all the things you have to get through today...you are just being lazy...this is not going to work for you anyway...what were you thinking? Whereas, my shoulder angel was kind and said things like: "Just give it a go...this is good for you...this is exactly where you're meant to be...just breathe...let your thoughts go...just breathe...you can do this!" Honestly, back then, those first ten minutes felt like an eternity of wasted time.

I'm guessing that many of you reading this can relate to my first experience of meditating and it being incredibly challenging, at first. Since I'm a pretty stubborn kind of person, I wasn't going to give up easily, and so I persevered. No matter how real the struggle and how vain the efforts seemed during those first few days of scary quietness, I pressed on.

And then something shifted. Not in a magic kind of way where I can now sit for hours and dive into total nothingness. No, I'm talking about a much more subtle transformation. Trust me, I am far from my meditation practise being an enlightened process, but the struggle has stopped. Now I can't wait to find this happy-licious space of mine where I can clear my thoughts and release things that do not support me on my journey to feeling and being the best, happiest, healthiest, most empowered version of ME. This new dimension is where I can let go of all my accumulated crap such as negative self-talk and old self-limiting beliefs. Instead, I fill this goddess zone—a space I was not even aware I had within me—with healing tranquillity, delightful inspiration, mind-blowing creativity, and incredible productivity. I feel surprised, every single time I meditate, by what flows out of me after I have given my full attention to breathing in the here and now.

I crave this time where I sit down like a Buddhist monk—sans orange robes—and with every breath, I touch base with my intuitive self and let go of my stressed, overly reflective, critical, and analytical self. In this infinite space, truly anything is possible. It is where this book was born. My life has not changed; I still juggle every single day the work of having my own business alongside the various challenges of being a mum. I would be exaggerating if I claimed that I'm never stressed anymore. I am still a doer, running around like crazy all day and who is in her mind a lot. But it seems I am much better equipped to deal with whatever life throws at me. My fast-paced life seems more selectively filled with purpose, as does my highly-strung mind. I feel that I can more fully tap into what I have to offer to the world by *living big* and by enjoying the moment more amid the chaos.

I wonder... "Were those quiet, mindful minutes a waste of time?" No, quite the opposite. I now know that there is no smarter or more effective way to hone into my endless potential, calm down my nervous system, improve my health, and throw out the window that extra belly fat I was holding on to unnecessarily. It is really quite incredible when you think about it. My career and business have soared to heights I couldn't even imagine possible. My relationships with my loved ones have never been more heartfelt and fully lived. I am not overstating it when I say, I feel like a much better version of the old me, and all this comes by simply allowing myself to mindfully breathe a few minutes every day!!!

Are you ready to try the same experiment and jump into meditation mode? I would so love for you to simply give it a go. You might find it much easier than I did. And trust me, it is so worth it. You do not require anything but your gorgeous self and a few minutes every day. Quiet consistency is the secret. Are you willing to unfold all your inner wisdom and magic? What are you waiting for, Gorgeous? Make time to breathe.

Benefits of meditation are:

- Balances hormones and stress levels.
- Lowers blood pressure.
- Improves symptoms of asthma.
- Reduces risk of cancer.
- Reduces systemic inflammation.
- Reduces risk of heart disease.
- Decreases symptoms of irritable bowel syndrome.
- Decreases anxiety, depression, and other mood disorders.
- Reduces overall tension.
- Lessens sleeping problems.
- Increases productivity.
- Heightens intuitive and mindful thinking over analytic and critical thought processes.
- Increases patience and tolerance.
- Increases self-awareness.
- Improves coping with stress.

FIND YOUR BREATHING, JOYFUL BEST SELF THROUGH YOGA

I believe nothing describes the art of practising yoga better than embarking on a journey of powerful self-transformation. I will be completely honest with you, yoga was a journey that took me a while to be fully ready to take. In hindsight, when I first started yoga, I wasn't aware of the amazing journey of growth and self-transformation on which it would take me. Initially, the athlete in me was in love with all those different poses and powerful fast flows that would make me sweat and increase my heart rate. There is nothing wrong with practising yoga this way, as long as you are able to stay connected with your breath and as long as you make it a flow of body, mind and soul. But, back then, I didn't. I was so focused on getting my asanas 'right' that I totally missed the point of true yoga. It's not about the perfect pose. In fact, every pose in yoga is perfect, when you connect with your breath and in doing so softly breathe calm and energy into the divine YOU.

Be gentle with yourself...yoga can be super strong. It definitely is for me. There are so many different forms of yoga to try out and fall in love with. There will be styles of yoga that will come easy to you and others that will be more challenging. I encourage you to be courageous and try out a practise that doesn't necessarily come easily to you so you can benefit from the growth. In my case this is Yin Yoga. Oh my gosh, I'm not lying when I confess to you that the first time I tried to let myself fall into full Yin, I had to succumb to this huge wave of feeling physically sick (like really-green-face, I-am-going-to-throw-up ill). Being unable to move while holding the pose is so intense and strong for my entire ME (body, mind and soul). I am naturally so much more Yang than Yin, so complementing this way of being with a bit more Yin is exactly what I need for more balance, even though not always very comfortable. I am not suggesting that it is necessary that you too, leave your comfort zone so far that you make yourself sick; this was just my journey. However, I do encourage you to be experimental and always have an open mind when it comes to your individual discovery journey with yoga. If you find that you are naturally more Yin, how about once in a while challenging yourself with a more Yang-inspired class?

Here is what else I love about yoga and what makes it so incomparably magical. In yoga, we will all always be students who are evolving and learning more, on so many levels.

- There is no perfect in Yoga; it is all about embracing the moment however imperfect this might show up in your practise. Yoga nurtures the mind, body, and soul. That is, it calms the mind and balances and revitalises the central nervous system while at the same time allowing our bodies to become stronger and more flexible.

- Yoga relaxes body, mind, and spirit. Certain Yoga poses, such as inversions where gravity is reversed and blood flowing back to the heart is encouraged, stimulate lymph drainage and freshly oxygenated blood flow.

- Certain yoga poses such as Tree Pose, Half Standing Splits, and Half Moon Pose, to name just a few, improve your physical balance as well as fostering inner/mental balance and enhanced focus.

- Yoga focuses on keeping your spine healthy and in alignment which improves posture and can reduce lots of back issues.

- Yoga boosts your immune system by encouraging lymph drainage and clearing of the respiratory system through proper breathing.

- Yoga boosts the detoxification process of your body (in particular, all those twists are great in cleansing right through the digestive system) and your mind (by being in the present and flowing from your heart, instead of focusing on your worries, stress, or ego).

Regular Yoga practise can alleviate certain health issues such as:

- Reduce high blood pressure.
- Reduce increased cortisol levels.
- Balance hormones.
- Improve bone density.
- Prevent cartilage breakdown by allowing joints to use full range of motion and therefore decrease symptoms of arthritis.

Yoga helps you to be more mindful which increases happiness and reduces anxiety, general worries and depression. It also helps you to be more in sync with your body, mind and soul which is a connection I feel we are increasingly losing, as our life becomes more automated and fast-paced. Living our life from a place of mindfulness can be advantageous in so many ways, including overcoming obesity and overeating.

So much has changed within me from when I first started my yoga practise. It is now my most intimate, sacred breathing space where I allow myself to fully be, falling in and out of the simplest poses, enjoying my connectedness to all that I am and my full presence in every breath of my flow. It is a place I so much want you all to find for yourself regularly. In one way or another, it is a place which feels like coming home to your best, most healthy-licious self.

PART 2:

YUMMY-LICIOUS — A WHOLE FOODS LOVE AFFAIR

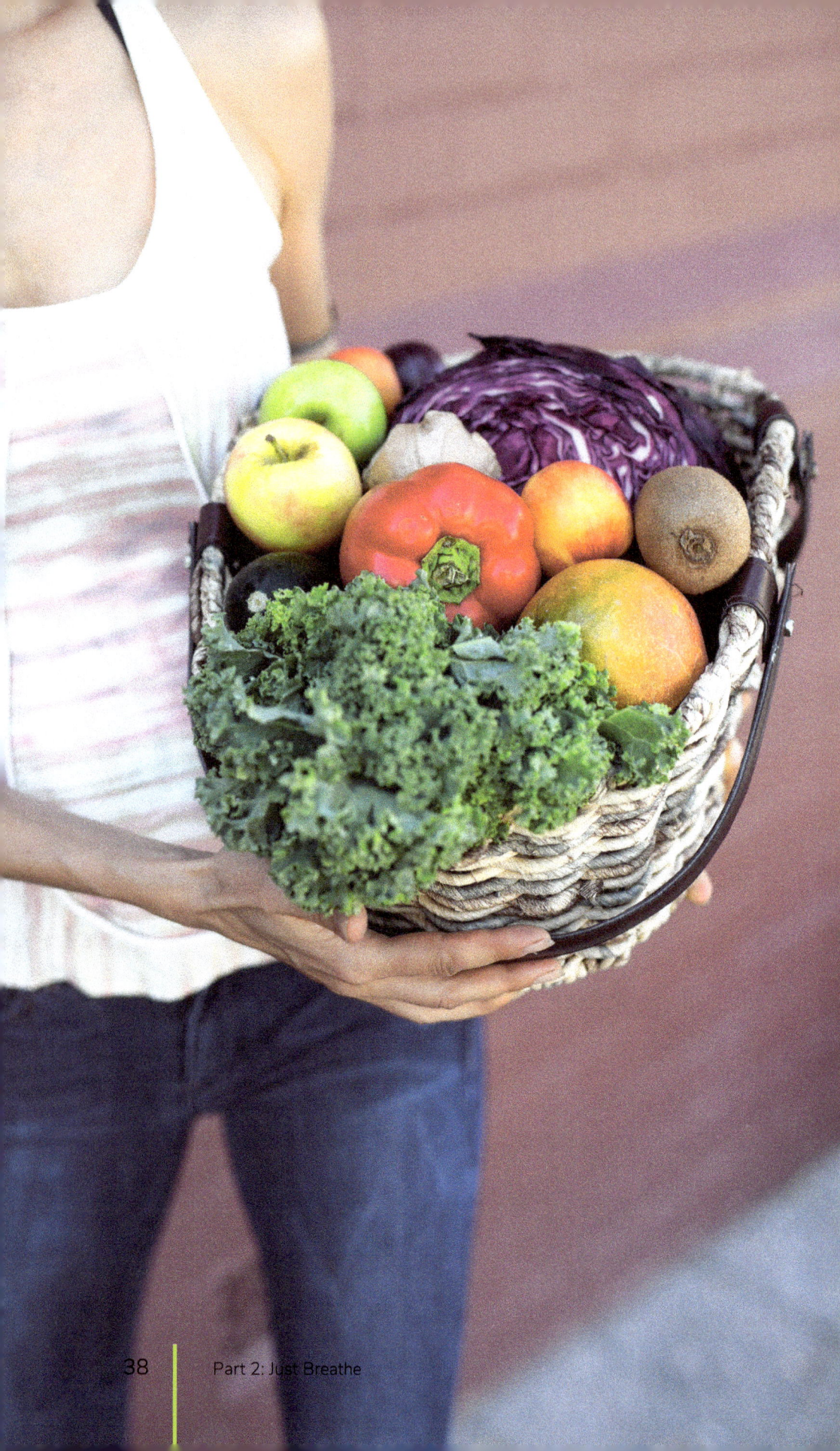

Part 2: Just Breathe

My Own Story

When I suffered a brain aneurysm at the age of 16 and lost control of my body, I had to re-learn everything. As I recovered, I promised myself I would always respect my body and nurture it with continuous, beautiful movement (exercise) in appreciation for having been given this second chance at life. I wanted to prove to myself, my medical team and my family that I was worth that second chance. What I completely misunderstood back then was the fact that health does not come only from moving your body regularly. It certainly is one valuable part in the healthy puzzle, but I learnt the hard way that there is something far deeper that makes me stunning and radiant. Without nurturing my precious self with the right fuel, all the best forms of movement and exercise could never uncover for me what makes me strong and amazing. This is what I want you to truly understand about your own precious self.

Keeping my promise to be the best, most healthy version of myself proved to be harder than I thought. I would be lying if I didn't admit that I fell off my healthy wagon more than one time along the way. Some falls were harsher than others and left me a little bruised at times.

In my early twenties growing up in Europe, I stumbled into the modelling scene. I suddenly found myself in this whole new world of glitz, glamour and so-called "perfect beauty." I was invited to dine with celebrities, movie stars and the super-rich (why are so many filthy rich men also super creepy?) I was also invited to take part in weird television quiz shows and, among other things, to showcase high end fashion by designers such as Versace and Ferree in their showrooms.

Even now, it sounds exciting and like a dream come true. I don't want to sound ungrateful, but as exciting as my new world of glitz and glamour was...was it really a dream come true? Maybe not! I pretty quickly realised that this outwardly glamorous modelling business is not so different from the meat industry. If you want to go far in the modelling world, you truly have to be prepared to do almost anything—lose 5 kgs in one week (even if you are already borderline underweight) or cut your hair in a style your client demands. You must be willing to alter yourself overnight by some arbitrary order, regardless of how the new version of yourself aligns with who you truly are or how damaging the instant transformation may be to your body, mind and soul.

It was a completely toxic environment for me, and bit by bit I spiralled deeper into this unhealthy world of thin-at-any-price where only your leg length, hip and waist circumference, and always your cup size, matters. The competition was fierce, and most girls I met or worked with were so committed to their dreams, they were willing to do almost anything to push me out of their way. To be honest, I never felt more unworthy and ugly in my whole life as I did at that time in that toxic environment. Due to the pressure put on me, I started training more and eating less. Because I didn't know better, I dove head first into establishing a very disordered eating pattern and body dysmorphia. I did not stop eating entirely, but it was very controlled, restrictive and governed by fat and calorie counting. My training amounted to sessions of self-torture. The deeper I got sucked in to this crazy world, the smaller my world became.

Not only did I totally lose touch with everything I believed in, but far worse, I betrayed my precious body day after day. Until one morning I woke up and decided I'd had enough. I felt horrible, weak, disgusted, unhappy, and totally and utterly unhealthy. I was the furthest away than I had ever been from the most radiant, healthy version of myself. I had tried to reduce calories so much and train so hard that there was not much left of my precious body.

Eventually (and thankfully) I realised this had to stop. I had to reclaim my healthy me again and find a way to reverse all of this. I made the most obvious decision: I quit modelling, a choice I have never once looked back upon with regret. I will not lie, though, healing my body, my disordered eating and relationship with my broken self was not as simple as turning my back on the modelling scene. It took me many years of self-exploration, tender self-compassion and nurturing kindness to understand that I was in fact, worthy of feeding myself with a wholesome, deliciously balanced and tasty diet which truly brings out the best in me.

With many small steps, one by one, I released self-limiting beliefs, healed my relationship with my body and with my eating. I feel that re-learning how to walk, read, write and think after suffering from the aneurysm was easy compared to learning how to love myself and treat myself accordingly. I guess this all goes back to a belief deep down within me which I held back then that I must feel pain in order to be good—that I must be punished to be worthy.

Interestingly, getting my power back to choose what and when to eat gave me a sense of deep fulfilment, a feeling I never was aware I possessed before. Unlearning such deep-rooted conditioning made room for more joy, more freedom and more self-appreciation.

It breaks my heart to see others battling against their bodies and being at war with their food. It doesn't have to be this hard. In fact, it can be really simple and so fabulously wonderful—if we only let it be or make it this way. Let's take charge together and start all over with our bodies, finding appreciation and affection for ourselves, no matter our weight or shape. It is really sad, but I have not yet met one single woman, whether she be a friend, client, colleague, or acquaintance, who has not tried one diet or another, or who has totally fallen away from healthy eating by developing one eating disorder or another. This has to stop, ladies!

Clarifying Food Confusion

Many of our less-than-self-nurturing eating behaviours stem from a whole lot of confusion about food. There are so many theories out there about how to best fuel your body to be your most stunning, healthiest self that we have forgotten to tune out the chatter and instead tune into our bodies and listen to what we truly need to out-glow ourselves, to feel absolutely amazing and to live a long, glorious life.

Fact: We are all different! It makes sense that what brings the best out in one person might totally not be the same experience for another. Yet we seem to think we can treat our bodies in the exact same way and get the same wonder-licious outcome, fully ignoring that we come with different shapes, different needs, different genders, different ages, different genes and ethnicities, different activity and strength levels, and different lifestyles. This type of thinking is clearly delusional! Do you take up learning the flute just because this is your neighbour's favourite hobby? Do you opt for soccer just because it's your hubby's favourite thing to watch and do? Do you assume pink as your favourite colour because your daughters do? Do you? I hope not. I hope you are designing your happy life according to your very own preferences, needs, values, beliefs and background.

It is just the same when it comes to nourishing yourself with healthy-licious foods. No, going paleo or becoming a raw vegan does not work for everyone... or at least not over a prolonged period of time. This fact must feel terribly frustrating! I get it. We long for clear-cut methods for success because after all, it helps make us feel safe and secure. It is less intimidating, and it is a whole lot less work. However, when it comes to food and nourishing your body, it simply does not work this way.

Your body is not a machine where you can simply rely on somebody else's experiences or successes, pushing yourself into the same cookie-cutter form. This may be seen by some as complicating their eating journey, but it also makes it so much more fun. I would argue that it's all a matter of perspective: Once you get the hang of hearing, seeing and listening to your own body's signals again, there is nothing easier and more exciting than nourishing your beautiful self with wholesome goodness.

Although there is no one way of eating that fits for all, there are a few principles that can help guide you through finding your most healthy-licious self.

HEALTHY-LICIOUS TRUTH 1: WHOLESOMENESS

Choose foods that are as wholesome as possible, meaning foods that are as close to their original, freshly-picked-from-mother-earth state as possible. Whole foods are full of beautifying and health-boosting nutrients such as vitamins, minerals, antioxidants as well as awesome phytochemicals like carotenoids and flavonoids. It is exactly these wonder-licious substances which allow our bodies to thrive. These nutrients nurture our bodies, beautify us and boost our health in ways we'll never be able to fully understand. There is nothing that can compare in terms of their magical powers for our well-being. This has to do with the complexity of compounds in real, unprocessed foods; that is, they do their magic by working synergistically together. No supplement can compare to such glorious alchemy, nor is the body able to use it anywhere near as well.

It's time to return to eating vegetables, fruits, whole grains, different forms of protein (plant-based and animal-based, if you would like) and fats[1] that do not clog arteries.

1 monounsaturated, polyunsaturated fatty acids; essential fatty acids, particularly omega 3 fatty acids

ACTION STEPS FOR CHOOSING WHOLESOME FOODS:

1. Avoid packaged and pre-cooked foods as often as possible. (No, you don't need to become a master chef. That would overstretch most women's time, not to mention their nerves, including my own! Instead, I am referring to ready-made packaged foods.)

2. Do not eat anything your grandmother would not recognise as food.

3. Check the ingredient list on the package. The longer the list, the more certain you can be that the product has lost nutrition, despite any healthy marketing claims on the package.

HEALTHY-LICIOUS TRUTH 2: VARIETY

In order for you to be your healthy, glowing, vibrant self, it is essential that you nurture your precious body with as many different whole foods as possible. The idea is to include a wide range of all three food groups in your healthy-licious diet, including wholesome carbohydrates, protein that brings out your best, plus satisfying good fats. The different food groups do different things in your body, and they all have their own special purposes. If you cut out one or more of the food groups, you run a big risk of your body (and with that, your health) falling out of alignment.

So, let's talk about those bad boys in the room, shall we? Carbs have received such a bad reputation over the last few years. Do they really make us fat and sick? Are they truly the devil himself? Of course not. It is true, though, that carb quality does matter. Yes, processed carbs found in all the white flours, pasta, breads, biscuits, etc., do not really nurture us. It is pretty hard for our bodies to tell the difference between the sugar in white foods and the sugar in lollies. The body responds to both with a quick sugar high and then a quick sugar and energy fall. We soon become hungry again and are more likely to overeat and crave all the wrong foods.

However, the story changes completely when it comes to complex carbohydrates such as your sourdough whole grain bread, whole grain pasta, brown rice, etc. Our bodies do need carbohydrates. But to truly thrive and glow with health they need the right kind of carbs. Processed carbohydrates make us fat and sick. Those complex carbohydrates, however, equip us with long lasting energy, beautiful skin and slim waist lines. Did you know that carbohydrates are the only fuel for our brain and the preferred source of energy for our muscles? Which means, if you deprive your body too much of healthful carbohydrates such as whole grains, fruits and vegetables, you will feel more and more weak and lethargic, your muscles are not able to perform as well and you might feel less clear and focused.

In addition, and I unfortunately see this all the time in my clients, eating too few healthful, beautifying carbohydrates actually leads to weight gain due to the quantity of fat and protein required to make up for the missing carbohydrates. As if this was not already frustrating enough, it also leads to increased cravings followed by bingeing on all those "forbidden" foods. This produces a result directly opposite of what you were hoping for.

To be clear: there is nothing at all wrong with eating healthy carbohydrates. They are full of slimming and gut healthy fibre plus many other nutrients our body needs. It is more about which carbohydrates you decide to nourish your body with which will make all the difference in your healthy-licious life.

Variety does not end there. Within every food group, there is a wide diversity of choices. For example, don't always eat only broccoli or kale; mix and match your veggies as much as you possibly can. Each colour of vegetable or fruit holds different minerals, vitamins and other phytonutrients vital for our well-being. Our body needs as many of them as possible. If, for example, we always eat only quinoa, we compromise our health with a limited array of micronutrients. Meanwhile, it also increases our exposure to any less favourable substances that are attached to it. Remember: No single food is totally free of by-products. We really don't know (in large amounts or accumulated over time) whether these can be toxic to the body. So, instead of eating mainly brown rice or mostly sourdough wholemeal bread, I suggest that you try lots of different whole grains.

ACTION STEPS TO ADD MORE VARIETY INTO YOUR WONDER-LICIOUS LIFE:

1. Always buy, cook, and eat as many colours of the rainbow as you can find.

2. Try not to eat one particular food, such as pasta or quinoa, on more than two (maximum three) of your seven days. Get creative and come up with alternatives to your usual staples. Mix up quinoa with teff, amaranth or buckwheat; switch your usual whole wheat bread to rye or spelt; swap spinach leaves for kale or for dandelion greens and so forth.

3. Challenge yourself to buy, cook with, and eat at least one food per week that you are yet unfamiliar with. I know this can feel like venturing out of your "I-know-what-works-for-my-family-and-how-to-get-it-on-the-table-super-quickly" comfort zone, but eating this way will not allow you to grow further on your journey towards your most amazing self.

HEALTHY-LICIOUS TRUTH 3: INDIVIDUALITY

It always surprises me that so many people seem to think even though we look totally different, live different lifestyles, have different tastes and habits as well as completely different backgrounds, ethnicity and genetic make-up, that we can all follow the same diet to achieve one and the same successful outcome. How do we come to even consider such a bizarre notion? Maybe we long to categorise things, to put them into different boxes so we can pull out the correct ones and push back the wrong ones. Our bodies totally do not work that way.

What our body needs is individualised nurturing. We thrive if we listen. Of course, a very active 30-year-old gym-going woman has very different needs from a 50-year-old sedentary office worker with a family history of heart disease. This is obviously a challenge when catering to the different demands and requirements in a family household. It's likely that your husband will want and need to eat differently than your teenage daughter or your three-year-old toddler, not to mention your own preferences. This bit can be tricky! However, it certainly does not require that you prepare four different dishes. That would only horrendously elevate your own stress levels, which is definitely not aligned with supporting your best self.

Do not despair; hear me out. Even though most of your family members might have different needs and tastes, everyone can still share the same meal. There is nothing wrong with making a generic meal of brown rice, vegetables, a salad, and tofu as an example.

You can cater to everyone's individual needs when it's time to dish up. For example, your husband will naturally have a greater need for protein and healthy carbs than you do, unless you are very active and fit. This is because generally, men have more muscle mass than women, which is metabolically active and needs to be fed. If your husband is regularly exposed to second-hand tobacco smoke, he has a higher need for vitamin C, too. If you have a family history of heart disease or cancer, you want to make sure you dish up extra plant and antioxidant super-powers with every dish. Your teenage daughter will need an even bigger portion than your husband (especially if he is not very active) to supply her with everything she needs while she's developing and growing so quickly. In order to satisfy your daughter's body's demands, sprinkle the larger portions with nuts, seeds or cheese or all three for extra energy. As for your toddler, of course, she or he wants plain foods in line with the latest allergy recommendations and will need far smaller servings of your meal.

I am a big fan of Buddha Bowls where you can add on or take away to everyone's taste. I also think that having healthy sauces, fun condiments and hot side dishes sitting at the table are great ways to bridge the gap of individuality. They make it possible for each member of the family to spice up their meals according to their tastes without your ending up a crazy, stressed cooking mess.

ACTION STEPS FOR TAILORING YOUR DIET TO YOUR INDIVIDUAL NEEDS:

1. Cook and prep your meals buffet style so they can be assembled according to individual needs.
2. Keep your main macros simple and then add on according to taste and requirements.
3. Do not go overboard with accommodating everyone's needs; there is a fine line between supporting others to thrive and making room for excuses.

HEALTHY-LICIOUS TRUTH 4: BALANCE

I feel this is the one principle most people struggle with. We all know, logically, that balance must be good for us and, in one way or another, we are all striving for it. However, too many of us have forgotten what true, healthy-licious balance looks, feels and tastes like. Nourishing your precious self in a balanced way means embracing the three different food groups so that they can bring the best out in you. That is: you do not experience any blood sugar lows or spikes, irritability, fatigue, unexplained mood swings or gut issues. Instead, you feel amazing with lots of good energy.

Just to clarify: I am not saying that you should be eating equal amounts of all three food groups (which might be useful under certain circumstances for some individuals, but more commonly will not be the case for most of us). Exactly what amounts of which food group is right for your personal journey, life, and situation will vary for everyone. The best way to know how much is right for you to achieve balance is by getting in tune with your body cues of satiety, hunger and fullness. I will dive deeper into what makes us overeat and how to overcome such habits in chapters 3 and 4 of this part of my book.

Creating such wonder-licious equilibrium in your body also means choosing foods which will keep your blood pH alkaline, not acidic. This means moderating foods that create acidity in your body, such as foods derived from animals, processed foods, sugary foods, alcohol, coffee, soft drinks, etc. An acidic blood pH makes your body far more susceptible to chronic disease; it has been linked to an increased risk of cancer, and it lowers the body's amazing ability to detoxify and renew its cells. Our body thrives on healthy-licious plant foods. We need to nurture ourselves predominantly with beautifying, natural plant-based foods to help keep our blood pH alkaline. You may choose to enjoy animal-based food or other more acidic forming foods, but only if they enhance your magic glow. It is essential not to overdo it with these foods, though, since they can make the body's pH tip over into less healthy acidic levels.

Finally, in discussing balance, it's important to not slip into a total black-and-white, good-or-bad, or all-or-nothing form of thinking. After all, it is important to enjoy your food. Your healthy-licious meal should leave you feeling pleased and satisfied, both physically and emotionally. Embrace and love every bit of your healthy diet! If you have favourite foods or dishes that you know aren't healthy and you still want to enjoy them, give them a space that is 20% or less of your diet in a week. If you fill the other 80% of your diet with eats that nourish your precious self, you can easily handle the other 20% without unreasonably increasing your risk for disease or weight gain. It is far healthier to wholeheartedly enjoy your wine, chocolate bar, white bread or pasta once in a while without any guilt than to deprive yourself of the little pleasures. If you end up feeling restricted and deprived, you are very likely to react with bingeing on exactly the foods your mind obsesses about.

ACTION STEPS TO KEEP YOUR BALANCE:

1. Eat from all the 3 food groups in amounts that bring the best out in your body (not because you have read that it is good to cut out carbs and eat more protein and fat).

2. Do not go overboard on acid-forming foods; **do** make sure you balance your blood pH by including lots of alkaline-forming foods.

3. Instead of shame-causing limitations, practise the 80/20 rule for healthy/fun balance.

HEALTHY-LICIOUS TRUTH 5: PLAN FOR SUCCESS

As we have already affirmed, changing your habits can be hard and can feel overwhelming, especially when those old habits are linked to limiting beliefs and/or are deeply ingrained over many years. The busier and more stressful your life, the harder it will be to put additional effort into your new, healthy-licious lifestyle. However, you can make your life a whole lot easier by setting yourself up for success from the beginning.

Set aside time each week, when you are full of positive energy and feeling enthusiastic, to prepare your healthy-licious food for the week. You may set a menu plan, organise your shopping, chop and organise your vegetables and prep cooking/storage. This will facilitate a quick and easy time in the kitchen on a day when you might otherwise feel you don't have the mental or physical energy required to plan and prepare a meal. This can be the victorious difference between feeling stuck and unable to accomplish healthy cooking and just getting it done. I believe this truth is the one that can really make or break your victorious journey.

To create wonderful success on your journey, it is super important that you cut yourself some healthy slack. Do not strive for self-manipulating perfectionism and do not look at making things more complicated than they have to be. Eating and cooking healthy-licious does not mean you have to cook up super complex, time-consuming, expensive dishes. *Simple is good*, and getting back to good old-fashioned basics is wonderful. For example, eggs are cooked in less than 5 minutes and are one of the most nutritious foods available. Thrown in a Buddha Bowl with steamed or baked veggies, salad leaves, lentils or chickpeas and brown rice can taste like a chef d'oeuvre. It is a truly simple dish that involves little time and no stress to prepare.

Finally, in order for you to set yourself up for awesome look-good-and-feel-even-better success, I invite you to become a label reader. This is not to find out how many kilojoules or calories you are eating. Counting calories is neither an empowering nor healthy and balanced way to choose your food. Reading labels is about knowing exactly what you are about to put in your mouth and digest in your body. I am a big fan of making informed decisions about how I govern my yummy life. So, when I invite you to join me in the label-reading club, it is to help you pay attention to ingredients that can quickly overwhelm your body. Unfortunately, the processed foods of today are loaded with toxic ingredients. I want you to take back control and be able to recognise these foods for what they are. Do not blindly trust packaging that falsely claims to be healthy or good for weight loss. Instead, turn your package around and make an informed decision by reading the ingredient list. Know that the ingredients are listed from greatest quantity to smallest, so pay extra attention to those first 3-5 ingredients listed.

I encourage you to look for these ingredients on your food labels:

Watch out for:

A. Unhealthy fats:

- Hydrogenated – trans fats
- Saturated fats – aim for those that contain less than 3g of saturated fat per 100g[2]

B. Hidden and added sugars:

- Other names for sugar – sucrose, dextrose, fructose, maltose, glucose, syrup, malt extract, modified carbohydrate, etc.
    - o 4.2g of sugar = 1 tsp of sugar
    - o WHO (World Health Organisation) recommends to eat no more than 5-9 tsp of sugar per day
    - o Dairy – contains about 4.7g of sugar from lactose (so subtract 1 tsp from your sugar balance)

C. Salt

- Other names for salt – baking soda, sodium bicarbonate, yeast extracts, stock cube, monosodium glutamate
- Avoid products that contain more than 400mg of salt per 100g

D. Preservatives, fillers, anti-caking agents, genetically modified produce, monosodium glutamate (MSG)

NB Always choose foods that contain at least 3g of fibre per 100g

FOOD PREP: ACTION STEPS TO SET YOURSELF UP FOR SUCCESS:

1. Try to lose your inner perfectionist and embrace a good-enough attitude towards yourself.
2. Sit down and create a menu plan for your week. (This plan does not have to be super detailed, it is more about knowing what to buy and what different meals you will cook – you can still decide to swap things around on the day if you would like to.)
3. Do a big shop for your entire week including loads of fresh fruits and vegetables, beans, legumes, pulses, wholegrains, nuts, seeds, healthy fats, and protein like eggs, yoghurt, lean meats and fish, if using.
4. Keep it simple and easy! Healthy does not mean complicated!!!

---

2 *except for dairy – this has to do with carbon chain length, i.e. those between 12 and 16 increase cholesterol; those over do not appear to do so*

- Purposely prepare a larger batch of food for your evening meal; fill your lunch for the next day straight away into a smaller container or jar and store in the fridge. This truly must be the easiest, most economical, most yummy-licious and healthiest way to ensure your body gets everything it needs despite you being so busy. Best of all, this doesn't take much of your precious time or effort.

- Extra bonus: Reserving part of your evening dish for the next day will help you control your portion size. For this reason, though, be sure to pack your lunch portion straight away into the fridge before you sit down to eat your evening meal.

5. Commit to a big prepping session on the weekend—it's so handy to have healthy-licious snacks ready to nourish yourself when hunger strikes or your blood sugar drops in the afternoon. Bliss balls, seeded whole meal breads, fruit loaves or homemade muesli bars will have to be some of my favourite ways to kill those afternoon lows. I also like using the weekends to fill seeds and nuts into little reusable zip bags or hand-sized containers.

6. Find the time in your day, whether in the afternoon or evening, to take the storm out of your mornings and organise all your meals for the next day. I don't know about you, but my mornings are always frantic, so having everything ready to go is totally vital for my entire family's survival—and I mean that!

- Cut up your fruits, place into containers and pop into the fridge.

- If you are having muesli, prep your overnight oats.

- Have your kale already cut and safely stored in a little container to throw into your eggs in the morning for a quick breakfast.

- In terms of lunch, I always make sure I have a big bowl of different sorts of lettuce and cabbage with spring onions in my fridge so that I can then fill them into smaller containers mixed with my protein, whole grains and healthy fats ready for the day's lunch.

- If you keep your salad dressing separate, i.e., you don't dress the whole bowl of salad, nothing gets soggy and wasted.

7. Take back control and become a label reader (watch out for refined sugar and its alternatives, salt, unhealthy fats, preservatives, genetic modified produce, monosodium glutamate, fillers and anticaking agents).

HEALTHY-LICIOUS TRUTH 6: SKIP RESTRICTIONS

The very sad truth is that most of us deeply believe that in order to be healthy or thin we must diet or restrict ourselves. I would like to challenge your thinking here and argue against it. First of all, where is the logic anyway? Restrictive dieting makes no sense at all. How could anything that deprives us lead to a positive, long-lasting, transformative outcome such as living in a body you love?

Any type of growth or lifelong success can only come from a place of abundance and love. Right? So, how can we expect fabu-licious results in regards to our health or weight by practising unkind, restrictive measures to our precious bodies, souls and minds? This equation will obviously not end in our favour. And yet, we keep believing this is the only way to go. We keep cutting out foods or even entire food groups. We reduce our nutrition down to mere figures as if our bodies were machines—as if putting a certain amount of kilojoules into that machine, called body which would then produce the so-called perfect body. Too many of us labour under the awkward impression that our bodies should function in accordance with this simple equation: fewer calories in than out equals weight loss. Unfortunately, or should I rather say, luckily for us, our bodies are much more complex than this.

It seems more than ridiculous. Let me tell you: I am done with all this dieting nonsense and my world has never been richer, healthier or more expansive, free and fun. I want this for you, too. Let me shout it from the rooftops: "Diets don't work, people!" Not in the long run, that is. If you are after quick results and are happy to dive into a world of yo-yo dieting or putting double the weight on after you have stopped limiting your eating, coupled with low self-esteem, then of course, by all means keep at it. But this book is not about that because I do not subscribe to that way of thinking. I am all about empowering and supporting you to live in a body you feel wonderful in, that feels amazingly vibrant, radiant and totally magnificent FOREVER. It is this kind of awesomeness you cannot bring about by forcing your body to do something it is actually not comfortable with.

So, let me give you the facts: diets don't work because our bodies are too smart. When we restrict our calories, our bodies adjusts by burning fewer calories, lowering the rate of metabolic activity. True physical magic, wouldn't you agree? So, this means that in order to lose more weight, you have to restrict your calories further and further, which is not very sustainable. Eventually, your body will have had enough of all this deprivation and will fight back. Your need, desire and urge for food and calories will be so strong that all of this barely eating will totally backfire and result in you eating more than you should and probably, on top of it, all the wrong foods. This isn't because you are weak or your willpower is not strong enough, it's because your body is trying to keep you alive and do what's best for you— always. Surviving on only a few calories per day is obviously not what brings the best out in you. Your body knows this; on this point as well as many others, your body is so many steps ahead of you. I would even go so far as to argue that dieting brings out only the worst in you.

Let me say it again: "dieting does not work." This is not only my very own painful experience, shared by my desperate clients (and others worldwide) who feel they have tried it all with no success, but research backs me up on this, too. As the language itself implies, going on a diet means that eventually you will have to go off it, so it is not sustainable in the long run. What happens once you stop with your crazy calorie restriction and counting? Not only will you put (very quickly) all those kilos back on, you are very likely to put on more fat than you had before because your body wants to outsmart your unfortunate circumstances and wants to see you covered against this famine you are apparently experiencing. Thus, it down-regulates your ability to burn fat and up-regulates your hormones that cause you to eat more. If this was not enough, all these unwanted, painfully gained, new fat reserves on your body bring nagging feelings of guilt, a self-esteem that just took a beating, and self-worth that just plummeted to a new depth. Needless to say, all this negativity is not exactly going to foster greater self-love, self-acceptance, positive self-talk or any other healthy thoughts and behaviours. You would have to agree, that is a pretty ugly and depressing cycle.

In summary: diets are effective in establishing an unhealthy relationship with your precious self and ineffective for long-term weight loss, vibrant awesomeness, and feeling wonderful in your beautiful skin. The whole concept of dieting is faulty, and it is about time we passed this knowledge on to our friends, neighbours and most certainly to our children. I dream that our next generation grows up knowing how to nurture themselves, the healthy-licious way. I want them to feel good about their wholesome, balanced diet without ever giving another thought to self-deprivation or crazy restrictions.

MY FOUR TRUTHS ABOUT DIETING

CAN HELP YOU EXTRACT
YOURSELF FROM POOR
THINKING AND DAMAGING
PRACTISES:

1. Diets slow metabolism.

2. Diets lead to yo-yo weight loss/gain.

3. Diets cause more weight and fat gain.

4. Diets create an unhealthy relationship
with yourself, negative self-image,
poor self-esteem and have potentially
devastating psychological side effects,
including eating disorders and body
dysmorphia.

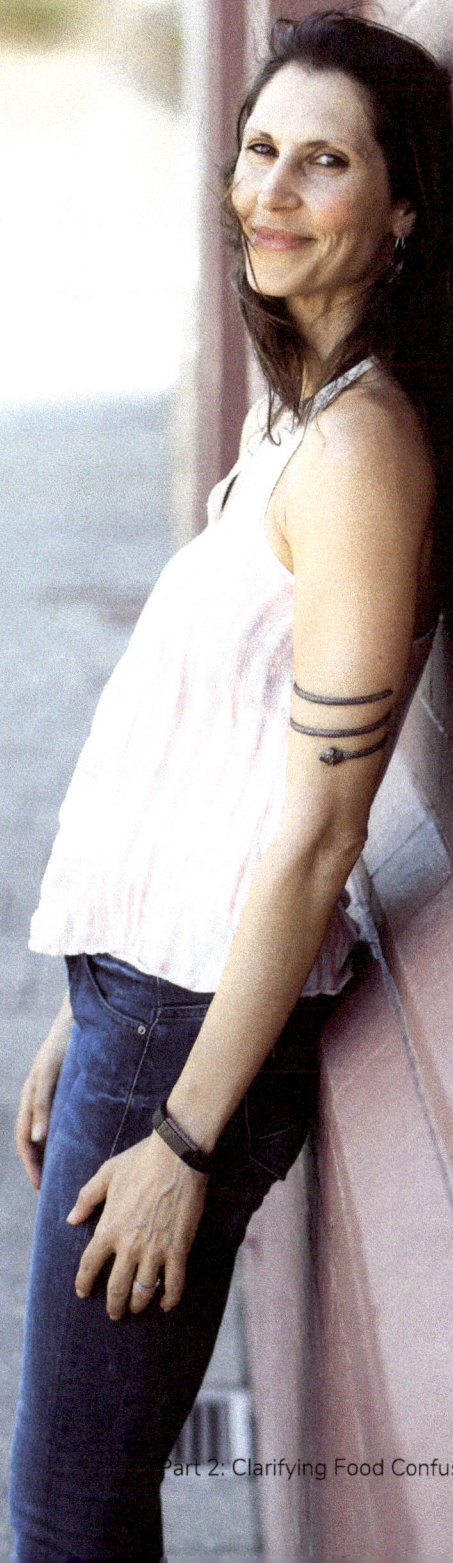

Abundant Life and Self-Compassionate Weight Loss

Are you wondering, "If diets don't work, what does? Is it possible to lose fat or weight from a place of abundance and self-compassion instead? And how does this translate into practise? Obviously, those extra kilos will not simply fall off me just because I have decided to love my body and myself more. "Or will they?" No, they will not. But if you are willing to love yourself unconditionally and treat yourself accordingly, you will also want to nurture your precious body and not hurt it. This translates eating into fuelling yourself with what brings the best out in you, both from within as well as from the outside. The fabulous news is: The same foods that do exactly that will also take care of your waistline, naturally.

REPLACE HIGH-CALORIE FOODS WITH HEALTHY-LICIOUS, NUTRIENT-DENSE WHOLE FOODS

Here comes the totally fun part! If your goal is a healthy-licious, slim body that you feel insanely amazing in, then all you have to do is go back to nurturing your precious self with health-boosting, nourishing, beautifying whole foods—foods that are bursting full of nutrients and are relatively low in calories, rather than high calorie, nutrient-deficient, processed junk foods. Yummy-licious whole foods do not trigger overeating or cravings. They fill you with satisfying micronutrients and gut-healthy, slimming fibre.

REPLACE OVEREATING OR EMOTIONAL EATING WITH MINDFUL EATING

Have fun with your wholesome produce. Do it in a mindful way by being fully present with all your senses while you eat. Turn off your mobile phone, put aside your tablet, newspaper or book. Turn off the computer, TV or radio and pay attention to what your food looks like, how it smells, and how the different textures feel in your mouth. Chew each bite properly while you place your cutlery aside your plate. Once you have swallowed that morsel, pick up your utensils again to prepare your next bite. Be mindful after each spoonful to check in with yourself whether you are feeling fuller and satisfied. Slowing it right down is good. The slower you go, the more present you are, and the more present you are, the more you become in touch with your natural cues of hunger, satiety and fullness. It can take up to 20 minutes for your body to realise that you have eaten enough and send the right signals out to your brain telling you to stop eating. Have you ever raced to swallow great spoonsful of delicious food only to realise too late that you have overdone it and you have gone beyond feeling comfortably full? I have, and it's not a nice experience to feel that uncomfortable, especially because such bouts of overeating also trigger feelings of guilt and shame, making it hard to be kind to yourself. If you practise slowing down your eating, you are far less likely to overeat.

As you learn to listen to your body, you will find that soon after you swallow and begin digesting your food, a first wave of fullness gently warms your being. It is really soft and your stomach is not very much extended at that time. It's crucial that you listen very carefully, especially if you are used to gulping down large amounts and filling your belly until you feel very full. This first wave is a message from your body that tells you that you've consumed the right amount for your energy needs.

This is such powerful information for you to know so that you can guide your eating experience. Of course, I am not commanding you to immediately stop eating at the first signs of satiety. However, if you know this simple truth, you can choose how much more you want to eat after you have given your body what it needs to thrive and be satisfied. There is nothing wrong with adding a spoonful here or there for your soul, the yummy-licious taste, and pure pleasure of eating as long as those extra spoonsful don't cause stomach cramps, bloating, indigestion or any type of negativity in your body.

EAT REGULARLY AND MORE FREQUENTLY INSTEAD OF TRYING TO EAT LESS BY DRAGGING OUT MEAL TIMES

Have you ever tried to drag out your meal times as a measure to eat less? I have, and I see it in my clients all the time. Our dieting mindset comes up with such creative, but ineffective ideas. Let us remind ourselves again to lose such thinking because it won't help lose the weight or change body composition. Instead, it will make blood sugar levels plummet...the longer you go without food, the more they will go down and as a natural response to blood glucose dives, you will crave all the wrong foods. You know the foods I mean, the ones that are full of sugar, unhealthy fats, other nasties and lots of empty calories without any of the beautifying, health-boosting goodness.

During this type of cycle, the body is crying out for a quick surge of dense energy. It's often incredibly difficult, if not impossible, to resist the body's urges. If this was not already bad enough, considering the fact that what you are actually trying to do is lose weight or reduce the extra fat in your body, you will end up eating larger portions when you are so hungry. If you had simply had a little healthy snack in between you could have saved yourself the anguish and extra calories that you ended up putting into your body.

I invite you to put concentrated effort into planning and keeping regular meal times each day. This can feel like another leap of faith and very different to everything you have been trying to do so far, but your old ways have never worked, so go for it! I know for a fact that feeding your body every 3 hours with a nourishing meal or a little healthy snack will help your body to trust that it is not in a famine. In return, your body becomes free to burn fat more easily, rather than clinging to it to help you survive an attack. I invite you to commit to not skipping any meals, ever again. The only exception to this is when you are truly sick, with no appetite because your body is focused on producing antibodies for your healing.

In practise, this means having breakfast every morning, ideally within one hour of getting up. If you are not much of a breakfast person, you can also split your breakfast bowl into two halves and only have a few bites or spoonsful and then save the rest for your morning snack. Having this first meal in your day is vitally important to give your body all the right messages. In other words, eating breakfast lets your body know that the night fast is over and that it can ramp up its metabolism again as it prepares you for the day ahead.

Next up on the menu is your morning snack. This is probably the one snack that is easiest to have without causing blood sugar issues. I urge you to make morning tea part of your most healthy-licious life. I am not talking about a huge feast here. Just nurture yourself with a little nourishing snack that catches your blood sugar from dipping down and keeps your metabolism fired up. Obviously, what your morning tea will look like will differ widely from one person to another. I, for example, am a very early riser and am active straight away so by 10 am I need to fuel my body with a decent morning snack. However, I know that many of my clients who get up later and are less active are very content with just a big cup of turmeric latte or a matcha latte, for example.

Lunch will ideally follow two to three hours later. Be mindful not to fall into the trap of keeping your lunch super small. It is important for you to know that you will not trick your body's metabolism by eating less. It will overcome small lunch sizes by claiming it all back with a large dinner. That said, dinner is not the time to make up for most of the food you missed out on during the day. Oversized dinners create gastric upsets followed by poor sleep, which in turn creates hormonal issues that can lead to further weight gain.

Not only that, large meals consumed late in the evening tend to more easily pile on those extra kilos since we often follow dinner with a relaxing, inactive evening. This part of our day is super important for our overall health, but not efficient in terms of burning extra calories. When we lay down to rest, our bodies do, too. Instead, be sure to have a decent size lunch which truly satisfies you, refills your energy stores and prevents you from overeating at dinner time.

After lunch, afternoon tea is probably the most important snack to avoid cravings, mood swings and blood sugar crashes. There are many factors that cause us to feel like we are running on empty once mid-afternoon strikes. It may be helpful to know that such afternoon crashes are part of our circadian (sleep and wake) cycle, but they can be greatly intensified by unbalanced hormones or riding the blood sugar roller coaster. For this reason, avoid refined sugar, coffee, alcohol or unhealthy fats in your afternoon snack. I recommend snacks that contain natural sugar with protein like fruit with nuts and seeds or nut butters. These are great pacifiers for cravings and for balancing blood sugar.

For many of us, dinner is the favourite meal of the day. Dinner tastes like another hard-working day done and a reward for everything you took on and achieved that day. It tastes like enjoying some quality family time and sharing about your day with your loved ones. It tastes like a well-deserved rest.

I get it, and I want your dinner to be full of all those different tastes of love, togetherness, fun and peace. But if your goal is to feel wonderful in your beautiful body again, which might mean you need to lose some weight, I want you to be mindful to not eat until you feel you have satisfied all of those feelings. Your dinner is there to be shared and enjoyed, yes, but the purpose of food is to fulfil and satisfy you physically, not emotionally.

Remember: Commit to eating your meals, at minimum, every three to four hours.

REINVENT HOW YOU FILL YOUR PLATE

Most of your success in exchanging a body that feels foreign with the one you were always meant to have is linked to your being back in tune with YOUR body's needs. Without becoming too prescriptive, I want you to regard the following suggestion on how to reinvent your plate as a loose concept which you will then tailor to your own individual needs, goals, life-situation, and make-up. These can look very different from one reader to the next, so please take this on in a way that suits you best.

In order for you to nurture your beautiful self with as much healthy-licious goodness as you possibly can, I invite you to divide your typical plate in the following ways:

Fill half of it with vegetables, greens and salads (when I say vegetables, I am referring to non-starchy vegetables such as broccoli, spinach, cauliflower, courgette, cucumber, etc., not potatoes or sweet potatoes).

Fill one quarter of it with different forms of protein (be sure to include at least half of your quarter with plant-protein here such as beans, legumes, tofu or other soy derived products, spirulina or other forms of seaweed, chickpeas, avocado, etc.).

Fill one quarter of it with whole grains, starchy vegetables or pseudo-cereals such as quinoa, buckwheat or amaranth.

Garnish your plate with about a thumb-sized source of healthful fats such as extra virgin olive oil (rich in heart healthy monounsaturated fatty acids) or sprinkle with nuts and seeds (those rich in omega-3 fatty acids) such as hemp seeds, chia, ground flax seeds or walnuts as well as other polyunsaturated fatty acids like those found in sunflower seeds, pumpkin seeds and almonds.

REPLACE ALCOHOL WITH DRINKING MORE H2O

For many of my clients, their hard day's work ends with a celebratory glass (or bottle) of wine or another form of alcohol. It is a habit that marks the time for shutting down and relaxing. However, if your goal is to change your body composition, shed some extra weight or become the healthiest, most glowing version of yourself, this habit does not align with your intentions.

I'm not saying you can never drink; enjoying your favourite glass of alcohol can be made to fit into your healthy-licious life if this is important to you, but not as a daily routine. The problem with alcohol is that it's very high in calories in return for almost no nutrients. (Red wine, high in the antioxidants, resveratrol and thiols, is the exception.) Furthermore, alcohol commonly increases appetite while decreasing inhibitions and good judgement, the perfect storm for overdoing those healthful portion sizes and choosing all the less nurturing foods. Research also shows that alcohol decreases metabolic activity while making you feel drowsier and more lethargic. Also, since alcohol is viewed by the body as toxic and potentially life-threatening, it will stop whatever it has been doing—such as digesting foods—in favour of metabolising the poisonous intruder, alcohol, first. For you, this means that as long as alcohol is available in the body, your blood sugar will stay low because your body is busy saving your life by processing the alcohol in your blood first. In addition, most alcoholic beverages are very high in sugar which increases your calorie intake and will cause even more havoc with your hormones and blood sugar levels.

Lastly, alcohol is a diuretic which means you will have to go to the bathroom more often with the result of your body being more prone to dehydration. In practise, this translates into your being thirstier with impaired judgement, leaving you more likely to confuse this thirst for hunger. This already happens too often, even when not under the influence of alcohol.

If you are after some great results on your journey towards feeling and looking the best version of yourself, I invite you to make alcohol part of your 20/80 percent rule and only include it on those special occasions where you very consciously and without any nagging guilt in the aftermath, include alcohol into your healthy-licious life. I would also like to invite you to make it as a little rule of thumb of yours to enjoy a drink after you have eaten and not before—to preserve your judgement of which foods to choose and how much to eat. Ideally, give your body an hour or more to start its digestive processes before it gets busy processing the alcohol.

Alcohol in a glance:

- Alcohol metabolism is given preference over any other food or drinks— putting digestion onto hold and keeping blood sugar low.
- Alcohol stimulates appetite.
- Alcohol reduces inhibitions and good judgement.
- Alcohol is high in calories and often in sugar.
- Alcohol is a diuretic causing your body to be more easily dehydrated which increases the risk to confuse hunger with thirst.

But why swap alcohol with H2O and not anything else? Did you know that your body is only able to burn off fat from food and drink or stored adipose tissue if your cells are supplied with enough water to make this lipolysis possible? And here comes the interesting bit from my point of view: water is vastly available and usually costs us very little, if anything at all. Drinking water as a step in your weight or fat loss journey is also extremely easy to do and so very beneficial. Other than actually getting off the couch and sweating your heart out, drinking water requires little of your precious energy or time. Right? Yet, most of my clients really do struggle with drinking enough water until they have retrained themselves to do so.

Let me help motivate your inner camel and boost your water intake.

1. Water helps you flush out waste products from your body.
2. The more re-hydrated our cells, the more effectively we can break down the foods we eat and the better we can absorb and assimilate them.
3. Fully re-hydrated cells do not confuse thirst with hunger and therefore we are much less likely to develop cravings.
4. Drinking enough water keeps your appetite in a beauty-licious healthy range (not to confuse with drinking water to curb hunger, which I do not recommend at all).
5. Nurturing your precious self with sufficient water throughout the day keeps your digestive processes going and minimises bloating, gas and constipation.

GIVE YOUR FAVOURITE FOODS A NUTRITIOUS MAKEOVER

I truly love eating, and I especially love eating healthily! I love how it makes me feel. It equips me with long-lasting energy, it gives my mood a happy boost and gives my impatience a makeover. And, it has to be said, I also love it for the pleasure. I am a very sensory person and I love eating foods that look appetising, taste delicious and make me feel good about myself. Yes...these three can totally co-exist. For you to truly lose this restrictive mindset of dieting and become super successful on your new healthy-licious journey, it's incredibly important that you create such space for yourself. A space where you get enormous pleasure out of eating nourishing foods that bring the best out in you, both from within and from without.

I invite you to give your most cherished junk foods a healthful makeover. Not because you can no longer have them, because you absolutely can if you truly want them, but because creating and enjoying delicious, beautifying and health-boosting food is so much fun! Give your favourite food vices a 20% share of your diet and they won't overtake you. To be successful on your journey, it is essential that you enjoy your food.

I confess, the first 21 days in particular of your transformative journey can be a challenging adjustment to your new tasteful life. You deserve to know that all those processed foods have dulled your tastebuds, making it a challenge initially to savour the entire blissful taste explosion whole foods have to offer. Your palate has been in overdrive by excessive salt, sugar and fats that trigger the release of stress hormones. That is so harmful! The process of rediscovering your natural tastebuds varies in length for everyone. Typically, you can expect this reset to take about 21 days. In that time, you may not find your new changes to be altogether delicious. Perhaps you might approach this with curiosity, like a child, exploring a wonderful, new world. I encourage you to back yourself because it will be totally worth it—because after all, YOU are worth it!

To ease your transition, consider the following:

- Gradually reduce your salt and sugar intake, rather than going cold turkey.

- Mix it up. Introduce new options by degrees to give yourself time to adjust to new flavours and textures. For example, to replace white rice with more healthy grains, start by cooking with half a cup of white, or half a cup of brown rice and half a cup of quinoa.

- Use lots of spices and herbs to replace the sugar and/or salt for added flavour. In particular, cinnamon, cardamom and nutmeg are great spices for hastening the switch.

- Include sufficient sources of healthy fat such as salmon, avocado, nuts, and seeds and if you use dairy, full fat Greek yoghurt.

- Gradually replace sugary soft drinks. Begin with a glass filled with half water and half fresh juice. Change the ratios daily, increasing the water and decreasing the juice, until you add just a spritzer of lemon juice or have fruit infused water.

- Keep things crunchy—texture can help a lot when bridging the taste gap from artificial to natural. Consider replacing your chips with crunchy nori sheets, homemade spicy roasted chickpeas, raw seeds and nuts, etc.

CONSIDER MORE PLANT-BASED PROTEINS OVER ANIMAL-BASED PROTEINS

I expect you are fully aware of the filling effect protein has on your precious body. Therefore, it is essential that every healthy-licious meal or snack contains a wholesome source of protein. However, just because protein is great and can be an important part in your journey to feeling and looking your best self again, this does not mean that more is better.

Unfortunately, some of the latest fad diets suggest replacing carbohydrates with great quantities of fat and protein to hasten weight loss. My view is, this isn't good. I confront this misconception *all the time*! It drives me crazy to find my clients desperate and fundamentally flawed because their diets have failed them. They have been trying so hard to do all the "right" things and have been eating "so well" only to gain more weight. The truth is, our bodies need just a little protein to feel amazing and function well. If we overfeed ourselves with protein, especially animal-based protein, our bodies become ever more acidic. This overwhelms all the digestive and metabolic processes of the body and this acidity, driven by excessive protein consumption, literally weighs us down.

I invite you to eat a more balanced meal consisting of wholesome carbs, healthy protein and fats. Adding more plant protein into your diet can be a bit of a magic bullet when it comes to weight loss and fat loss. While meat, particularly red meat, takes a very long time to make its way through our digestive system (up to 72 hours to fully digest red meat), plant protein is digested fairly quickly. Not only that, it is full of soluble fibre.

Soluble fibre mixed with water forms a gel. Research suggests that this not only contributes to reducing belly fat, it also acts as a natural appetite suppressant. It down-regulates hunger hormones, such as ghrelin, while it up-regulates hormones that make you feel full. It sounds almost too good to be true! Those plant proteins filled with large amounts of soluble fibre also taste insanely amazing! Triple win! What are you waiting for, Gorgeous? Add more of those marvellous legumes, beans of all sorts and chia seeds onto your plate in exchange for animal-sourced protein. I promise, you will not regret it!

REPLACE LARGER SERVING DISHES WITH SMALLER ONES

When you have fallen out of tune with what your body needs to feel wonderful, you have usually also lost your sense of judgement for how your portion sizes creep up over time. It can feel rather tricky and overwhelming to reduce those portion sizes back to amounts that allow your body to thrive, especially when you are trying to replace patterns of deprivation and restriction with kindness and an abundance mindset. For you to feel satisfied with your meal, the appearance of a full plate is quite vital. Research backs this up. When you eat a full plate of food, you usually feel satisfied. The interesting bit is that it doesn't appear to matter if you're eating from a large plate or a smaller one. As long as the plate looks full and you get to eat all of what is on that plate, you feel a sense of blissful fulfilment—excuse the pun. While your body struggles to know how much food you truly need to have had enough and while you are still at risk of overeating, it can be incredibly helpful to simply exchange a large dish for a smaller one. Feel free to take this one step further—trade your big spoon for a small one and do the same with your fork.

Cravings and Different Forms of Hunger

Cravings are powerful, and being able to manage them plays a major role in you successfully losing weight. We commonly crave foods that are bad for us; this often leads to extra bites being added upon already-full stomachs, resulting in guilty shame and even embarrassment. To top it off, we often then feel like a failure. That is totally the opposite of what I want to achieve with this book. Therefore, it is my mission to empower you with information and knowledge about those undeniable urges to eat certain foods. You deserve to take back control of your happy, balanced healthy-licious life. Trust me, there is a life beyond food cravings and it feels pretty amazing and wonderfully free.

WHERE DO FOOD CRAVINGS COME FROM?

Experiencing food cravings is a sign that something in your body, soul or mind has fallen out of balance. Before you begin blaming yourself, please understand that this is not your fault. I want you to know that the more belly fat you carry, the stronger your cravings can be. This fat around your middle wants to be fed and usually it is not asking for kale or quinoa. It has its own very strong physiological response, so if you have doubted your willpower and talked down to yourself for being weak, stop right there. Your cravings have nothing to do with your willpower and no, there is nothing wrong with you. However, there is everything wrong with the food industry that conspires to capitalize upon the physiology of cravings. I would love to believe that the food industry really has our best interests at heart, and that these big food labels with their concerns are here to bring out the best in us—to nourish us from the inside out. Unfortunately, there is too much evidence to the contrary.

Did you know that food manufacturers hire food scientists to design food products with hard-to-resist flavours and textures? They are paid to discover our pleasure points and bombard them with these irresistible flavours and textures. They are keenly aware of the fact that people react strongly to MSG, sugar, fat and salt. They understand fully that we humans develop irresistible cravings, even addictions to these ingredients. In my world of healthy-licious happiness, this is very uncool, and, in fact, it makes me sick just thinking about it.

Let's dive deeper into the different versions and causes of cravings or "hungers" and learn how you can take empowered steps towards a balanced life, free of cravings.

SUGAR HUNGER

One reason for your cravings is that the food industry adds sugar to almost everything...and not just a little here and there. It is added in vast quantities, and in the most creative ways, to just about everything. Whether it is salty, sweet, or sour, it's likely you are consuming far more of this sweet, sugary poison than you are even aware of. The human body is not built to metabolize sugar in such overwhelming doses. Since your body always has your back, it does its best to manage all that refined, white powder as it can by releasing more insulin into the bloodstream. Eventually though, something has to give...and unfortunately, it is your health. Due to your body being under enormous stress, attacked by horrendous quantities of glucose in the bloodstream, it has to suffer.

Please understand, this is not a call to entirely eliminate refined or added sugars from your diet because this is unrealistic and unnecessary. However, I do want you to be able to make informed decisions on how much sugar you consume and for you to know exactly how sugar affects you. And lastly, I want you to know that you can bring sweetness to your life with more wholesome alternatives.

The Many Faces of Sugar

Sugar takes many forms. This discussion focuses on refined, simple sugar. It is what is added to your favourite dessert, cake, pastry, ketchup, boxed breakfast cereal, flavoured yoghurt, lollies and any other processed foods—for example, white flour, white bread, white rice, etc.

All these highly processed carbohydrates have the same effect on our bodies—a high spike of blood glucose followed by a sudden crash of blood sugar levels. Your teeth might be able to withstand the sugar for a time, but your precious body will undoubtedly suffer.

A tiny little bit of chemistry

Hopefully, a simple chemistry lesson at this point will not be too dry and uninteresting but instead educational and inspiring. I would like to share with you a basic understanding of what simple sugars are made of and how different sugar units can trigger different responses in your body. Chemically speaking, simple sugars are either monosaccharides—meaning they contain only one sugar molecule which can be either glucose, fructose or galactose. Or, they are disaccharides, which means they contain 2 sugar molecules such as is the case in lactose (or also commonly referred to milk sugar), sucrose (our typical table sugar) and maltose (other common food sweeteners such as malt syrup). Lactose is made of the sugar molecules galactose and glucose; sucrose is made of glucose and fructose and maltose is made up of two glucose molecules.

Sugar sources high in fructose include:

- Sucrose (table sugar)
- High fructose corn syrup
- Agave
- Honey
- Maple syrup
- Coconut palm sugar

The body's cells use glucose to produce short bursts of energy. Any of the simple sugars not immediately used for energy are stored in the body; however, our bodies have a hard time metabolising the fructose molecule that comes from refined sugar. (Naturally occurring fruit sugar in fresh produce is metabolized differently). The only organ that is able to break down fructose is our liver which turns it into fat. Obviously, the more fructose you put into your body, the busier and more burdened your liver becomes. Sadly, this abuse of our livers often results in fatty liver disease which closely resembles a liver diseased by alcohol abuse. In addition to removing toxic substances from our bodies, the liver has additional and essential tasks to perform. It regulates metabolism, processes and assimilates nutrients and deals with fat accumulation. A liver compromised by too much fructose cannot effectively perform these tasks. Suffice to say, sugar causes more turmoil and distress to our precious, once-goddess bodies.

Let me empower your understanding with a list of how sugar can damage your body:

- *Inhibits the body's immune system.*
- *Causes obesity.*

- *Upsets the balance of vitamins and minerals.*
- *Causes hyperactivity; interferes with concentration and learning.*
- *Causes irritability in children.*
- *Causes "sticky blood", heart disease and high blood pressure.*
- *Disrupts fertility.*
- *Speeds the ageing process.*
- *Causes acid indigestion and malabsorption in the digestive tract.*

Sugar has a scary-huge impact on your immune system because without a strong immune system, you are bare and defenceless. Your body is well equipped to deal with small bouts of high blood sugar, but is pretty vulnerable when it is constantly flooded with an unending assault. Not surprisingly, as your system's defences slow down, the more desperate and hopeless your body's ability becomes to combat against the glucose. The result is increased systemic inflammation. This inflammation is linked to an increased risk of heart disease, cancer, high triglycerides, obesity and high blood pressure. Not only that, all those sugar surges are driving your poor pancreas straight into irreparable burnout. Without a healthy pancreas, you are headed towards diabetes, obesity or metabolic syndrome. Not so sweet, after all.

It has been suggested that such oxidative stress in the body leads to shortened telomere length in the body. The shorter those telomeres, the faster the process of cellular ageing. This means excessive consumption of sugar not only hastens disease processes and lowers our life expectancy, it also gives us wrinkles. I do not know about you, but for me, sugar is a deal breaker!

YOUR BRAIN AND SUGAR

Sugar is highly addictive. The reward centre in our brains, the mesolimbic centre, lights up on sugar just like it does with drugs. Sugar sends a flood of happy, feel-good chemicals like dopamine and opioids into the bloodstream. As with other addictive drugs, we feel awesome, happy, comforted, and/ or excited. It's a very fast lived *high*, though! The problem with sugar, unlike heroin or cocaine, is that it's legal, affordable, easily obtained and socially promoted. However, it too comes at a high price when it comes to our health.

After the sugar rush and excitement comes the downward sugar crash, leaving you heaps worse than before. Adding guilt to the mix due to the poor food choices doesn't soften or ease the downward spiral, either. Even worse, every sugar *high* increases your tolerance to the sticky poison. You will have to consume more of it the next time to get the same feel-good kick. As you can see, it's certainly not a good cycle to be in.

The concept of individuality truly applies to every single piece of your overall health puzzle. When it comes to your receptors for happy chemicals, it is important for you to understand that some individuals are far more sensitive to sugar than others and, as a consequence, they crave or feel sugar withdrawals more acutely. I am one who is more sensitive to sugar. That sticky-sweet poison used to have a pretty tight, ugly, controlling grip on me...but I am pleased to say, not any more. I am done with living my life *not on my own terms*. I want to be the best version of myself and feel healthy and strong and in control of my healthy-licious life. To do this for myself has meant dropping all unhealthy relationships with sugar.

Sugar increases risk of depression, anxiety and other mood disorders.

As if what I've just shared with you wasn't enough, excessive simple sugar consumption has also been linked to increased risk of depression, anxiety and other mood disorders. As mentioned before, a diet high in simple sugars causes systemic inflammation, slowing down the immune system to a very slow crawl. These inflammatory processes have a far-reaching impact beyond your physical form, spreading to a foggy brain and sugar-betrayed soul. Metabolic syndromes such as insulin resistance have been linked to compromising the communication in brain cells that are responsible for memory and learning. In addition, symptoms of depression and anxiety are made worse on the high-low blood sugar roller coaster.

But...there is more: humans have no enzyme in place that helps the body regulate fructose consumption. This means that when we eat foods high in fructose, our bodies cannot signal when it has had enough—there is no sense of satiety or fullness that naturally comes to our rescue. As an example of this, have you ever noticed how easy it is to over-eat on a bag of gummy-bears? Whereas, the same amount of raw nuts or 90 percent dark chocolate would have us feeling excruciatingly stuffed?

THIRST HUNGER

An adult body is made up of about 60 percent water, therefore, it's not surprising that water is vital for our looking, feeling and being our best. However, all too often we don't seem to recognise that we are thirsty and we need to drink more water. When we were young, we knew perfectly how to differentiate thirst from hunger, although as adults we are often confused. The reason for this is that both signals come from the same part of the brain and can look and feel similarly. We can feel very sluggish, dizzy, light-headed, or experience difficulties in concentrating, thinking clearly and focusing on whether we are actually thirsty or hungry. It is also important to note that by the time we notice thirst, we're usually already quite dehydrated.

Here are a few tips on how you can distinguish thirst hunger from food hunger.

Signs of thirst hunger:	Signs of food hunger:
Dry eyes, mouth and skin	Stomach rumbling
Increased heart rate	Stomach feels empty
Both	
Feeling sluggish	
Difficulty to concentrate	
Irritability	
Nausea	
Dizziness	
Headache	

Ask these questions of yourself to determine the difference between hunger and thirst:

- ❓ How long ago was your last meal? If you have eaten within the last 2 hours, you are more likely to be thirsty. However, if your last meal was 3-4 hours ago, your stomach is probably empty and asking to be fed.

- ❓ How much have you been drinking? What did you drink? If you have been drinking coffee, decaf, fruit juice, a high sugar drink, an energy drink, black or green tea or alcohol, you are very likely to be thirsty.

- ❓ When was your last drink of water? If you haven't been drinking at least 1 big glass of water or water alternative (such as an herbal infusion in cold weather) within the hour, you are likely to be thirsty.

ACTION STEPS TO TAKE TO AVOID CONFUSING THIRST WITH HUNGER:

1. Drink regularly—at least 1 big glass of H2O every hour. Drink more water if it's hot and humid, you're very active, if you've been sugary or salty foods, drinking sugary or salty beverages, or drinking alcohol or coffee.

2. If you're unsure whether you are thirsty or hungry, try having a big glass of water first and wait for 10-15 minutes. If your feeling of hunger subsides, you know your body was on the quest for water. If you still feel hungry after you have rehydrated your cells, you are probably hungry. Go and nurture your body with healthy-licious whole foods.

3. Hunger develops slowly. If your hunger came on more suddenly, it is likely to be more a craving than real hunger.

4. If you are truly hungry, you are happy to eat anything to keep your blood sugar and body happy. If you are experiencing a craving, you are after a certain kind of food.

EMOTIONAL HUNGER

Have you ever eaten a tub of ice-cream because you were unhappily in love or devoured an entire bag of crispy chips after eating a full meal? Have you ever rewarded yourself with that enticing piece of cake after a hard morning's work or sat down with a bottle of wine thinking you will have just one glass after a busy day? Yep, that is called *emotional eating* and it happens in response to our emotions rather than our body's needs.

You know what? Doing this once in a while can be actually part of your healthy-licious lifestyle, as long as you are mindful that you're soothing your emotions, and as long as you have other coping mechanisms in place as well. It is not healthy for you to soothe your feelings of anger, pain, boredom, sadness and frustration by eating and/or drinking. Emotional hunger tends to kick in much more suddenly, almost like an impulse that takes over us, as compared to true hunger for food. Hunger that is triggered by feelings is so much stronger and harder to resist than food hunger, which usually builds slowly and thus offers plenty of time to come up with wholesome solutions. The tricky bit is that you might not always be conscious of the fact that you're actually missing something in your life, that deep down there is something not quite right. The illusion that all is well makes it harder to see that you're eating to fill the gap, to bring sweetness or crunch to your not-so-fulfilling life.

So, are you eating emotionally? Ask yourself the following questions:

❷ Do I eat to make myself feel better; to calm, soothe or make my life more fulfilling?

❷ Do I feel out of control around certain foods?

❷ Do I regularly binge on junk foods until I feel over-full?

❷ Do I feel emotionally attached to my junk food eating rituals, almost like junk food is my friend? Does eating junk food make me feel safe?

❷ Do I regularly eat junk food which is then followed by feelings of guilt?

❷ Do I tend to continue eating, even though I am already full?

What are the differences between physical hunger and emotional hunger?

1. Emotional hunger comes on very suddenly and seems super urgent and almost over-powering, whereas physical hunger develops more slowly and only has the same urge once we have not eaten for several hours.

2. Emotional hunger cannot be satisfied with food. No matter how much you eat, you will never feel full by the junk food you put into your body. When you eat to feed physical hunger, you feel satisfied after you have eaten, even if the reaction is delayed.

3. Emotional hunger asks for certain kinds of foods, typically foods that stimulate our feel-good hormones such as the unhealthy fats, sugars and salt in junk foods. When you are physically hungry, the thought of an apple or nuts is just as appealing as junk foods are.

4. Emotional hunger often leads to bingeing on junk food in a frantic, uncontrolled manner. Physical hunger allows you to take your time to eat slowly and mindfully.

5. Emotional hunger happens almost spontaneously and demands immediate attention, while physical hunger allows for preparation and sitting down to eat.

6. Emotional hunger is often accompanied by feelings of guilt and shame. You will usually have an inner sense of how out of control this kind of eating is and that it does not nourish your body. This compounds the problem of emotional hunger.

The good news is...You can take back control and stop feeding your emotions with food. Be gentle and kind with yourself, though. Very obviously you are hurting from something, so make sure you are taking great care of the vulnerable you as you are transitioning from reacting to your triggers with junk food to nourishing your soul.

ACTION STEPS TO CUT EMOTIONAL EATING AND TO GET CENTRED WITHIN YOURSELF:

1. Get in touch with what it is you *really* need—what feelings you're trying to experience through eating the junk food. Are you feeling unhappy, angry, sad, anxious, nervous or bored? Also: Did you learn emotional eating as a child? Did your mum always reward you with sweets when you did something well? Or did she always bake you a cake when you felt sad? The more honest you are with yourself, the easier it will be for you to hit the pause button once you are triggered.

2. Check in with your soul whether you are feeling fulfilled or whether you are lacking something in your life. Get clear on what it is you need to put into or take out of your life to be happier and able to live your soul's purpose.

3. Whenever emotional hunger strikes, consider taking the following steps instead of putting something down your throat:

   - Take a walk.
   - Exercise.
   - Get a manicure, massage, etc.
   - Enjoy a hot shower, bath.
   - Spend time with friends or call a friend.
   - Practise yoga.
   - Meditate.
   - Learn something new.
   - Read a book.
   - Garden.
   - Paint.
   - Spend some time doing something you love and that has meaning for you.

STRESS HUNGER

When your body is subjected to prolonged sustained stress, its reaction is to release cortisol. Cortisol regulates your body's energy intake by selecting the most appropriate food needed for survival. It's no surprise that cortisol's first pick among the many choices available will most certainly fall to high calorie foods that deliver fast energy. To make cortisol even more powerful, it appears to also have a stimulating effect on our appetites by releasing more ghrelin, the appetite increasing, I-feel-hungry hormone, when stress levels are prolonged.

In addition, cortisol inhibits insulin production to ensure your bloodstream is flooded with glucose to power through the fast action required to either defeat the perceived attacker or to run away. All of this is, of course, super helpful if you are in an actual, acute situation of physical stress. It also makes perfect sense that you would try to replenish your blood sugar stores after physical exhaustion. However, when the subject is chronic stress, these physical survival strategies begin to bite you in the butt. If you react to stress as if you're fighting a lion or outrunning a tiger without doing either, the unsurprising consequences show up in your waist. That increased belly fat, however, adds more stress to your body, resulting in more cortisol production, resulting in more cravings for junk food which then just results in even more belly fat.

Arggh...what a frustrating cycle to be in.

ACTION STEPS TO MANAGE YOUR STRESS MORE EFFECTIVELY WITHOUT FOOD:

1. Organise yourself well.
2. Love and accept yourself.
3. Control your environment instead of allowing your environment to control you.
4. Nurture your gorgeous self with wholesome real foods.
5. Move your beautiful body more and in ways that bring out your best.

6. Practise relaxation techniques (e.g., deep belly breathing, meditation, focus on calming mantras).

7. Rest yourself sufficiently and regularly. Get some good sound sleep, take quick hourly breaks, allow time for your eyes to rest, create routines that allow your mind to rest in between daily challenges.

8. Listen to your body. Take seriously signals such as headaches, frequent colds, insomnia, heart palpitations, lack of concentration, irritability, stomach upsets, loss of appetite, constant appetite or hunger, exhaustion, waking up tired and try to address them promptly. Remember, your body is constantly communicating with you to bring the best out in you—do not ignore it! Instead, partner up with your body like it's your best friend.

9. Enjoy yourself. Make time regularly for having fun; schedule quality time into your busy schedule and treat it as though it's an important business meeting; the happier you are, the healthier and more fulfilled you will be.

10. Reward yourself with healthful, quality leisure time. Plan family trips you can look forward to, book yourself in for a massage, meet up with your favourite girlfriends.

EXHAUSTION HUNGER

Similar to stress hunger, when you are overly fatigued, your body secretes more hunger hormones (ghrelin) and fewer hormones that signal to us that we have had enough (leptin). Thus, the more tired you are, the hungrier you become. When perceiving stress, your body releases cortisol, lowering blood glucose levels and amplifying hunger. However, just because you feel hungry does not necessarily mean that you are burning more energy and require additional calories (unless you have dramatically changed your habits toward more exercise and movement). Your wonderful body strives to protect you and produce the extra energy needed to compensate for all the exhaustion and stress you feel, but the truth is, the energy you truly need cannot really come from food. When you feel overcome by debilitating weariness, you need rest. You need to sleep and carefully replenish your soul and mind. Next time you think about eating that bar of chocolate to give yourself a little boost of energy after a restless night, think again. Plan time into your schedule to rest.

ACTION STEPS TO HELP EXHAUSTION HUNGER:

1. Be extra mindful to avoid caffeine after lunch.

2. Be mindful that when you're tired, you're more likely to experience more cravings and feelings of hunger.

3. Nurture yourself with a warm cup of naturally sweet herbal infusion such as liquorice or cacao chilli tea (my personal favourite).

4. Eat even more fresh and wholesomely energising foods like raw vegetables, salads, small handfuls of nuts and seeds, sheets of seaweed.

5. Eat small amounts of cell nurturing whole foods regularly.

6. Take a power nap.

7. Use aromatherapy balancing and/or energising essential oils.

8. Take time to meditate, have a hot bath, a massage, facial or pedicure/manicure.

SITUATIONAL OR RITUAL HUNGER

Sometimes your cravings will be triggered by situations or habits you have created that are outside of you. Do you need to have dessert every night in order to feel fully satisfied? Is a night out without alcohol really a night out? Do birthday gatherings require creamy cakes and tons of lollies? Do you switch from work-mode into relax-mode by pouring yourself a big glass of red? Do you crave chocolate just because you know it is in the pantry? These hungers are very clearly based on either habits you have created or on situations you associate with certain foods.

The first step to overcoming ritual hunger is to get clear on what situations or habits trigger you. After that, you either remove your trigger or, if this is not possible, change your circumstance. For example, if you routinely pour a glass of wine after work, change your routine. You might remove yourself from that situation by creating a new routine when you come home. Make a commitment that instead of walking into the kitchen and pouring a glass, you find a quiet space in your home to sit down for a ten-minute meditation to clear your mind before tackling the rest of your busy world. Do this religiously every single day. The more often you do this the less you will associate "I have finished my working day and am starting to relax" with foods or drinks. Another approach to break the junk food/drink routine is to simply remove it from your home. If it is not there, you will not consume it. Substitute it with a healthy alternative, even.

Whatever you do, do not knowingly expose yourself to situations or routines that lead to mindlessly overeating all the foods you have decided to eliminate from your life. If your girlfriend with whom you usually eat cake calls, ask her to meet you for a walk. If after dinner must be punctuated with dessert, get up from the table, brush your teeth straight after and ring a friend. The impulse to respond to your trigger will lose its grip within 10-15 minutes. If you can find a bridge while the trigger subsides, the win is all yours.

SCREEN HUNGER

Do you have to munch on something while watching TV in order to complete your screen experience? Screen hunger has a power of its own. Again, check in with yourself. Be brutally honest. If you know that watching TV or eating in front of a screen derails your healthy-licious eating plans, then consider rewiring your TV-linked eating brain. Being in front of a screen is one thing and nurturing myself with food is another, and the two together are incompatible companions for healthy-licious eating. Take charge and enjoy some invigorating movement while you enjoy your favourite programs. Try push-ups, squats or crazy plank variations. Consider replacing the TV with a good book, or practise meditation whenever the urge arises to put something in your mouth. If you choose to munch, do it mindfully and with intention (that is not with all your attention diverted onto the screen, but instead fully focusing with your entire being on the process of eating). Remember, the snack is a snack only, and not feeding the ritual addiction. If you truly must have something to nibble or crunch on while in front of a screen, choose something that nurtures and honours your beautiful body. Try a soothing warm cup of naturally sweet infusion or raw veggie sticks instead of the mindless consumption of unhealthy fats-sugar-and salt-laden junk food.

CELLULAR HUNGER

For most people, cellular hunger is difficult to decipher. This is truly sad; cellular hunger is the natural hunger with which we were once all so perfectly tuned. Before our palates, brains, souls, and bodies were exposed to ideas and influences which led us to mistrust our body's innate wisdom, we had an insatiable appetite for foods that nourish and replenish our cells. Cellular hunger happens when you've existed on a narrow diet, restricting certain foods or food groups. It's characterized by misreading or distrusting your body's signals—you mistake thirst for your body's actual need for the nutrition of a cucumber, carrot, piece of nut, brown rice or avocado.

It is so tricky to recognise such body talk and respond to it appropriately because you have unlearned trusting your body. The diet culture tells you your body is wrong, that you cannot trust its greedy needs. Your parents told you to eat more than you wanted. Your friends make fun of you because you dislike coffee. No wonder you have become utterly confused and have trouble knowing which food calls to follow. The key to hearing and trusting your body cues again is eating mindfully. Ask yourself whether you are craving something cold or warm. Something creamy or crunchy. Something spicy or sweet, something to chew on or something to simply swallow. Ask yourself if there are any whole foods that come to your mind when thinking of such attributes.

What if you are craving ice cream and potato chips? That is not cellular hunger. Have a look again through all the other many different forms of cravings and hungers described above. Cellular hunger is different from all of them because its request is for whole foods filled with vitamins, minerals, and many other health-boosting, beautifying nutrients. The more, the merrier.

Overeating & Binge Eating: How Much Is Enough?

Too many of my clients struggle with knowing when they have eaten enough. It almost seems that part of growing up is losing that natural wisdom on how to nurture a body with healthy-licious foods in the right amounts. We somehow stop trusting our innate knowledge and start believing in what everyone tells us to do. Mum says, "finish your plate." The food industry targets their marketing to children and teens: "burgers, fries, and junk food—it is what the cool kids eat," and "how much can YOU eat?" as they parade an endless array of beautiful-but-false food across the screen. Chick flicks show girlfriends and their besties coping with life's heartbreaks by eating a big tub of ice cream. We get bombarded everywhere with ideas on what to eat and how much to eat. It is hardly surprising that overeating and binge or compulsive eating dominate this world of confused eating. We have forgotten that eating is our most basic form of self-nurture. We missed learning to respect our bodies by giving them exactly what they need.

Eating should be exactly this: no more and no less. And you know what? If you go back to eating no more and no less than what your body needs and begin nourishing your body with healthy-licious whole foods in a mindful way, all your issues of overeating and binge-eating will naturally resolve. However, I accept that with all the different messages overlying your natural wisdom, it can be quite a journey to uncover your raw, knowing, eating SELF again.

Your intuitive eating self is incredibly powerful, beautiful, kind, very truthful, and always reliable. While you are on your search for her, get ready for all the joy, liberating freedom, and capable skilfulness she will bring you. Once you fully welcome her back as your self-regulating angel, your relationship with your eating self will flourish to heights you never knew were even possible. As a welcome side effect (with sustained self-nurture, that is) you will know exactly how much your body needs to eat to be the best version of its most glorious, goddess self. You will lose those extra kilos. Binge and compulsive eating will become a vague, fading, unpleasant memory of your past.

Are you ready, my gorgeous friend, to embark on yet another healthy-licious ride with me? To uncover your inner body wisdom—this total eating goddess within you? Okay, let's do it then.

WHAT MAKES US OVEREAT?

I know from experience that it is neither fun nor easy to have a brutally honest look at the behaviours that have crept in over the years. However, seeing the way things truly are is the first uplifting step—even if it feels anything but uplifting in the first instance—towards the new YOU. Please remember to congratulate yourself again for opening your eyes wide, taking a deep breath, and simply going for it. You are truly wonderful and you can do this. So, let us have a closer look at all the things that can trigger overeating, in addition to the list of false hungers we discussed in Chapter 3. Overeating can cause you to lose a true sense of how much food you actually need to thrive and can trigger more food cravings. Being aware of what causes you to eat more than you need can be incredibly eye-opening and your first super-empowering step to taking back control of your healthy-licious body.

Some of this might feel and sound very familiar by now, whereas other bits and pieces might reach you as new information.

You tend to overeat when you:

- Engage in mindless eating. That is, when you're distracted by something else or your attention is not turned to the act of eating.

- Eat overly stimulating foods such as junk foods full of sugar, unhealthy fats, and salt.

- Are dehydrated.

- Are unaware of your exposure to external cues that stimulate your desire to eat something Such as commercials or foods you see and smell on pretty much every corner of every street... food has never been around in more abundance and as easily available as it is now.

- Eat compulsively as compared to a planned meal.

- Eat out of containers.

- Are stressed, overly tired, experience difficult emotions, or are bored.

- Deprive yourself of certain foods, causing more compelling cravings, setting yourself up to eventually inevitably overindulge.

- Have too many different tastes and food choices on one plate (depending on the food choices this does not necessarily have to be a negative thing). Research shows the more boring your food, the less you will eat.

- Are overly hungry, such as when your blood sugar is dipping too low because you are not eating regularly enough. Trying to skip meals will definitely backfire. You will make up for the skipped meal by eating double (or more) than what you would have eaten in that one go.

As mentioned before, I am not a big fan of giving you a rigid count of macros or calories or amounts of food at hand that you should eat. I know that in the long run, things will not work for you this way. What your body needs might be so different from what mine thrives on. Every body and everybody is different and has different emotional, physical and soul needs, plus we all have different ways of learning. We hold different values and beliefs and our eating behaviour was shaped by different experiences. It would be absurd if I applied my body's wisdom to yours, ignoring your own physical makeup and entire being. But don't despair. I know your portion size struggle is real and I will share with you a few simple strategies that bridge the gap between not knowing how much is enough to trusting your body's innate wisdom of hunger, satiety, and fullness again.

PRACTICAL ACTION STEPS TO GUARD AGAINST OVEREATING:

1. First and foremost, practise mindful eating. This truly is the most reliable tool when it comes to uncovering your most healthy-licious self.

2. Eat regularly. Never, ever, skip meals or snacks.

3. Avoid becoming overly hungry. Hunger is not your friend. When your blood sugar has gone too low, your body instinctively responds. You are driven to binge on unhealthy foods, ensuring you are protected against the next period of famine.

4. Eat foods that are high in fibre, high in nutrients, high in plant protein, and that make you feel satiated. (See the more detailed list of foods that help you get better in tune with your own body wisdom below.)

5. Drink enough water throughout the day.

6. Use smaller dishware. Research suggests that we feel a sense of fullness after eating a filled plate, regardless of the size of the plate, as long as it was full. By switching to smaller crockery, you can gently re-teach your body how much is enough.

7. Use serving plates and bowls that contrast well with the food you are eating. Some research suggests that the more our food blends in with our dishes the more we eat until we feel full. (Maybe the food blends in so well that we are less aware of how much food we are eating?)

8. Fill your plates in the kitchen, rather than serving family-buffet-style at the table. Just the effort required to return to the kitchen for more food will give you time to pause, tune in, and consider how full/sated you already are. It separates you from the act of eating for a moment relieving you from mindless, compulsive, automated eating. If nothing else, it will win you the time it takes to register the feeling of fullness.

9. Avoid trigger foods—high sugar, unhealthy fats, salt, and/or alcohol.

10. Avoid situations that you know will trigger your overeating.

11. Brush your teeth immediately after your meal to clear and neutralize your palate. This can help to reduce the desire to eat more.

YOUR BODY AS YOUR GUIDE

If you are still having trouble trusting your intuition, use your body as a guide on how much to eat:

Your cupped hand holds the just-right-for-your-body amount of wholesome carbohydrates, such as whole grain pasta, brown rice, sweet potato, or rolled oats.

Your palm matches the just-right-for-your-body amount of protein, such as eggs, meat, fish, and dairy.

The length of your thumb is the just-right-for-your-body measure of healthy fats, including nuts and nut butters, seeds, and various oils.

The size of your fist shows you the **minimum,** just-right-for-your-body, amount of vegetables, including broccoli, cauliflower, lettuce, cabbage, etc., that will nurture your body the healthy way.

FOODS THAT CAN HELP YOU TO FEEL MORE SATIATED:

1. **High-fibre foods**—specifically all the healthy-licious plant foods, e.g., barley, oats and other whole grain products, slightly undercooked or al dente whole-grain pasta, avocado...

2. **High-protein foods**—chickpeas, seaweed, tofu, chicken, eggs, avocado, chia seeds, quinoa, etc. Please note, I am not advocating protein-based meals or overdoing your proteins. Rather, make sure you always do include a healthful, nurturing source of protein with every meal (please remember, especially the incredible power of plant protein).

3. **Nutrient-dense/low calorie plant foods**—vegetables, beans, pulses, legumes and more vegetables.

If you have a pattern of over-eating, your body is accustomed to requiring large quantities of food to feel satisfied. Nurturing your body with these healthy-licious foods will create satisfying volume in your meals without adding more belly fat to your waistline. This is crucial for your success. In time, you can retrain your stomach to feel satisfied before it becomes painfully full. However, as is the case with every transformation, this will take many small steps of gently reorganising your body's perceived set points of feeling satiated.

OTHER THINGS AT PLAY WHEN IT COMES TO OVEREATING

Another shocking fact is that everywhere, our portion sizes keep growing. Don't believe it? Compare the size of a restaurant meal four years ago to how much is piled upon our plates these days. I am screaming in disgust! It seems that the wealthier we become in this global economy, and the greater the availability of such a wide variety of food, the more the food industry presses its agenda by supersizing everything. No wonder the western world has become so obese.

If we proportionally increased our physical activity and movement and if those big meals consisted of fruits and vegetables, with some whole grains and healthy fats, we might have a chance at outwitting this continuous overindulgence. But those things aren't happening. Our wealth and state-of-the-art healthcare are not making us better. Instead, we are becoming more unwell on so many levels. Obesity rates have never been higher, diabetes has never been more prevalent and sadly, heart disease, cancer, high blood pressure, and fatty liver diseases are more frequent in our communities around the globe.

Let's turn things around, my beautiful warrior girls. Let's not be fooled anymore by oversized drinks and meals when we eat out or order in.

DOWNSIZE THAT SUPERSIZE: ACTION-STEPS FOR SELF-NURTURE WHEN DINING OUT OR ORDERING IN:

1. Request the server to plate only half of your entree and to pack the remainder in a take-away box. Enjoy that for your next day's lunch or dinner.
2. Enjoy in twos: Request the server to divide a single entree onto two plates so you can share.
3. If you doubt the new portion size will satisfy you, order additional greens and salads.
4. Ask your server for a half-glass of wine or, ask for a 2nd empty glass and share with someone you love.
5. If you are worried a small glass of wine will leave you thirsty, request some more water instead of wine.
6. Divide take-away food onto two plates, instead of eating from the containers.
7. Instead of drinking high-calorie drinks or alcohol out of take-away cups or bottles, pour them into smaller glasses and save some for another time.

HOW SELF-LIMITING BELIEFS AND BEHAVIOURS IMPACT YOUR OVEREATING

Do you have a sense there is more to your eating habits and overconsumption than you've ever stopped to consider? Have you ever wondered why you feel so drawn to consume such vast quantities of food? Do you feel almost like eating this way is a self-fulfilling prophecy? Like you just know you have got to stuff endless amounts of foods down your throat to be and feel like YOU?

Have you ever considered that your self-limiting beliefs are at play here? And without this conscious awareness, you are constantly trying to live up to those beliefs, whether they're good or bad, whether they serve you or hurt you.

You are a divinely complex human being. While this is truly wonderful, it can also make your life so entangled, confused, and messy. Here I would like to explore with you the notion that your mind is divided into two parts—the rational mind and the subconscious mind. The conscious mind is very much in charge of the execution of all of your actions. You decide whether or not to eat this or do that. You choose whether you should stop eating now or to just go for another handful of those salty, crunchy bites. You could say *it is in your command*.

Your subconscious mind is filled with your beliefs and values. It accepts any idea that is pressed upon it repeatedly over time by the conscious mind. It does not have the power to judge whether a thought is true. It simply receives whatever is held continuously by the conscious mind and stores it as a belief. Once that has occurred, the subconscious maintains this belief as a template for the actions that reinforce it and it rejects any action that disagrees with it. This is good if the subconscious keeps only truth within it, but it lacks a truth filter. Only the conscious mind can decide if a thought or idea is true or false.

If the conscious mind decides to challenge a false, limiting belief, it causes a stressful condition that psychologists call "cognitive dissonance." Some people mistake the anxiety-producing discomfort of cognitive dissonance for a character flaw or a huge warning that something is about to go terribly wrong. This is where fear happens and it is where people mistakenly disbelieve that they cannot change.

Cognitive dissonance is simply this: It is changing your mind.

In terms of self-care and discovering your divine goddess strength and gifts, this is vitally important to understand. Recognizing that your subconscious mind is merely serving its protective function over you, you can lovingly and gently replace the old, limiting beliefs with new truths. Practised over time, you will truly change your mind about who you are and what you are capable of achieving. You will not need to wilfully force, shame, or punish your body into your perception of what it should be if only it were not so obstinate. Instead, you can bathe your conscious mind with your beautiful truth so that your subconscious learns to protect you with love. No more fear. No more shame. No more defeat. Just light and love.

Do you hold self-limiting beliefs? Do you carry ideas that, unchallenged, undermine your success?

WHAT ARE COMMON SELF-LIMITING BELIEFS?

In my daily practise as a Nutrition, Health and Fitness Coach, I find these common limiting beliefs playing havoc on my clients and students. They are very familiar to me, as I have personally had to undo them in my own mind.

- I am unworthy.
- I am a failure.
- I am not good enough.
- I am too weak and have not enough willpower.
- I do not deserve success... (to be thin, to live a fulfilled healthy life, to be happy, to be fit, to be loved, etc.)

Can you see how such limiting beliefs actually act as a road map of your life? If you believe you are unworthy of living your best life, of losing this weight or being fit, your subconscious mind will do everything in its power to make that true.

CHANGE YOUR STORY: STEPS FOR OVERCOMING SELF-LIMITING BELIEFS

Are you ready to manifest your deepest desires by overcoming such beliefs?

Ready, set, go! It's game on, Gorgeous! The amazing, all-is-possible future is yours.

Apply the most gentle, tender self-compassion and kindness towards your precious soul, heart, mind, and body:

1. Meditate. Spend some quiet time with yourself and ask your heart, "What do you believe about yourself and hold on to that keeps you stuck and from achieving your purpose?" Please listen because your answer is within you.

2. When a limiting belief shows itself, accept it with gentleness. Do not shame it—just receive it as it is. Greet it with a nod and a knowing hello.

3. Give love to your soul and body for being willing to hold that false idea in order to protect you from disappointment and pain. Thank it for keeping you safe.

4. Send loving thoughts to your heart and tell yourself that you are well and safe in your own keeping. That you no longer need that old idea to hold you safe and keep you stuck. That your soul can safely trust you to move to your true authentic self.

5. Take on that new powerful truth. Dwell on it even. Make it your magnificent obsession. Say to yourself "I love my body", "I radiate unique beauty", "I am enough now and always." (Now your turn, Gorgeous: Which loving thoughts about yourself can you add here?)

SELF-LIMITING BEHAVIOURS THAT CAN TRIGGER OVEREATING

Self-limiting beliefs interfere with your happy-licious, natural eating self, but did you know that many people have also adopted a variety of self-limiting behaviours that can trigger overeating? Let me share the ones I have frequently encountered in my practise.

▶ *Self-limiting values*

Sometimes self-limiting beliefs have their origin within your values. That is a bit of a controversial statement, I know. Unravelling the mystery of how your unseen values collide with reaching your goals is tricky. I mean, how can something good, like the morals and values you hold about the world, stand in your way? Well, they will if they are not fully aligned with your goals. You might, for example, believe in the virtue of hard work and believe that hard work alone makes success possible, and without a great effort, you do not deserve success. If your weight is transforming with little effort, that result does not align with what you believe about hard work and success. Therefore, you will subconsciously invent ways to make your weight loss journey difficult. You will start manipulating and sabotaging your best efforts, so to speak.

Have you ever started off a health journey only to find that things were going far better than you expected? What did you do? Most likely, you began anticipating the curveball that would prove you right, that weight loss has to be hard. And then what happened? The curveball came and you said to yourself, "See. I knew it. It could never be that easy."

I know it sounds almost ridiculous to look at it in such black-and-white terms. I mean, who would sabotage their best efforts and undo all their hard work for the goals they have worked so hard to reach?! Well, obviously no one would mindfully derail their progress, so if you find yourself acting in opposition to your goals, go inward and find the disconnect.

ACTION STEPS TO OVERCOME SELF-LIMITING VALUES:

Find ways to realign your values with your goal. If you believe that hard work is the only way to success and your new lifestyle feels actually easy, you might say instead that you believe that **good work** is what is necessary. It is certainly true that nurturing your precious body and mind with daily goodness is indeed **good work**. Not all good work is difficult, and not all difficult work is good. Check in with what you value and you may discover that your success actually aligns with your values and that your values do indeed align with your success.

▶ *Perfectionism*

Hmmm...it gets trickier. Trust me, I truly know what I am talking about here. Even today, I am still coping with my self-destructive, perfectionist tendencies. I constantly work on owning my flaws and irregularities. I practise daily, stepping into imperfect action instead of stopping myself over not being able to ever live up to my own unreachable expectations.

What perfectionism is and what it is not:

There is a fine line between very driven people, who strive for excellence and are willing to take constant steps to better themselves, and perfectionists, whose actions are motivated by an inner, critical voice. Those who strive for and achieve greatness have developed inner qualities, beliefs, and motivations that carry them from success (and failure) to success. They are willing to dig deep, to work hard, and to rise each time they fall.

Perfectionists are haunted by an inner voice of criticism. No matter how hard you try or how much effort you put into your project, it will somehow never be good enough. This is a dangerous place. The lies embedded so deeply in your subconscious destroy your work. When your inner voice tells you constantly that you are a failure, it robs you of feeling good about yourself and sabotages the development of a thriving, empowered relationship with your beautiful self. So, to cope with all that pressure you put on yourself, you develop coping strategies. Some people become brilliant at avoiding situations where their perceived weaknesses might be exposed. Then they fall into denying themselves the opportunity of being good enough, of growing, and of fine-tuning their skills. These elements of growth are huge milestones to success.

The fear of failure might make you constantly postpone the things you truly need to do to become the most powerful, glowing, happiest version of yourself. You are so convinced that you cannot deliver the way you expect yourself to, you would rather not try at all or put the brakes on your endeavours before the embarrassment or pain of not succeeding gets too overwhelming.

What does this all have to do with overeating? Well, it has a lot to do with it. If you are a perfectionist starting this lifestyle journey, you could well experience that your perfectionism shuts down the transformational tango of to and fro, of two steps forward and one back. When you discover that you cannot live up to your pie-in-the-sky expectations, you are likely to sabotage your endeavours altogether.

ACTION STEPS TO OVERCOME PERFECTIONISM

1. *Embrace and love your imperfections.*

    Think about it: what is it that you love most about your best friend, husband, partner, child? Yes, they have beautiful souls and hearts, but what makes them so lovable and special—what are their unique quirks? Would you agree that you do not love them for being perfect? Learn to look at your own imperfections through these same loving eyes.

2. **Be okay with making mistakes.**

   It is from every big and little mistake that you learn and grow. The more you are willing to make mistakes, the more rewarding your journey. It took me a long time to rewire my expectation that "I am not allowed to make any mistakes." I would sit over something I had written forever trying to perfect it, rather than risk people knowing I made an error. How does this help me on my mission to make this world a happier, healthier place though? It does not. So, little by little, replace "perfect" with "real." It will allow you to make your dreams a reality. Trust me.

▶ *Fear of Failure*

You don't have to be a perfectionist to have a paralysing fear of failure. Have you ever said to yourself, "I cannot do this because I am not smart enough?" Or, "My body just isn't made for that." Or, "I am not even going to try because I know it will not work for me"? Well, you just let fear of failure stop you. Instead of trying, you listened to your fear and gave up before even taking action. Again, this is something I have experienced firsthand and seen in my clients as well. It drives me crazy. Here they are—those brilliant, stunning, capable women walking through my door, believing their inner negative, devil voice of insecurity more than their own abilities. It is hard to say how many years they have wasted on playing small, tolerating being overweight, being unhappy and unfit when they have more than everything within themselves to become everything they have always wanted to be and totally live up to their wildest dreams.

Fear of failure is very real. You cannot simply brush it away and pretend it does not exist. But you can do something about it.

▶ *Fear of Success*

As confronting as it may sound, fear of success is just as common and potent as is fear of failure. It simply is the other side of the coin. If you fear success, you might feel really uncomfortable when getting close to succeeding in something. This fear might be associated with your parents telling you in childhood that you are a failure. Such traumatic past experiences may have instilled the belief in you that you are not worthy of success. The thought of success may also trigger in you the fear of disappointment or being exposed to high risks you cannot live up to or withstand.

ACTION STEPS TO OVERCOME FEAR OF FAILURE AND FEAR OF SUCCESS

1. Tap into a powerful memory. Can you remember a moment in your life where you felt incredibly fearful of something, but you somehow did it anyway? Can you remember how you felt after? Did it make you feel stronger? Were you proud of yourself for doing so? Remember the strength you felt then, and one action at a time now, follow your example.

2. Think back to a time where you succeeded in something even though you were afraid. Internalise how the experience filled you with a sense of pride and accomplishment. Deeply reflect on the boldness the experience gave you. Take that sense of empowerment and infuse it into your new situation. Push yourself to take action, come what may. I know you can do it. I know YOU will.

▶ *Learnt behaviours*

The way you nourish yourself with food, exercise and anything else is a great mirror of the relationship you have with yourself. Often this relationship is unkind, unproductive, uncaring, and unloving. Your relationship with yourself can sometimes be clouded with traumatic childhood experiences—things you learnt when you were a child and little; the memories held live deep down in your body. If your parents used food or any other substances as a coping mechanism, you are very likely to have internalised such behaviours and copied them without even thinking. You might have grown up with a mother who struggled with her own body image and as a result practised restrictive and binge eating. Maybe she made harsh comments about your body or your eating habits and made you feel badly about yourself. All of this might have led you to lose a positive connection with your precious body.

ACTION STEPS FOR ADDRESSING LEARNT BEHAVIOURS

1. Pay careful attention to your eating behaviours. A food diary might help you to make more sense of what is driving them. Be honest with yourself: How were you feeling when eating and how did the foods make you feel? Were you mirroring any behaviours you observed in your parents?

2. Get support on board. Learnt behaviours can be very hard to unlearn. Know that you do not have to do this all on your own. It can be very powerful to share your observed behaviour with someone you trust and invite them to hold you accountable to make step-by-step changes to such behaviour.

▶ *Overeating as a form of self-protection or punishment*

Obviously, how you treat yourself is entirely in your control. If you established an unhealthy, disconnected relationship with yourself due to past traumatic experiences, this might show up as self-hatred and a compulsion to punish yourself. Over- or under-eating becomes not only a form of rebellion against self but also instils a false sense of safety and protection. In your mind, you manage to avoid addressing your emotional pain by laying down protective layers of fat to cover your tormented, fearful, unlovable heart and soul. Undereating creates a thrill-inducing illusion that you have control over the situation—especially when it comes to your eating. Sadly, just the opposite is true. Control does not exist in this false cover of pride.

Where can you start changing your self-sabotaging story? Accept and love yourself totally the way you are!!! With kindness!!! Treat yourself with the same gentleness, open-mindedness, care and flexibility you are giving to others. You deserve it. In fact, you need it to thrive. You need it to tap into your true power and stop unhealthy cycles of over-eating.

ACTION STEPS TO ADDRESS SELF-PROTECTIVE AND SELF-PUNISHING PATTERNS

1. Go inward. Ask yourself if you are eating to numb your pain. If so, can you try and instead love your pain? I know this sounds a bit weird. I hear you asking: How can you possibly love your pain? Because your pain is a precious part of you. It makes you uniquely you. If you accepted it as exactly this, you might find a way to actually embrace it instead of trying to flee from it, which entirely disarms the power overeating once had for you.

2. Do you deserve to be punished? For what? And why? Recognise this pattern of belief is false. You DO NOT deserve punishment, not from outside of you and absolutely not from inside of you. Accept that you are not broken. Remember that "perfect" means being complete—and you are complete, just as you are. You have everything you need already for making your life what you want it to be. Repeat to yourself over and over, "I am enough. I deserve love for who I am now. I love myself and I love my body. I give my body good things and my body gives good things back to me. My body takes care of me and I take care of my body." Please make this your new daily mantra.

The Next Generation

As a mother of two gorgeous princess girls, this question shoots right to my heart: what about them? I know how frustrating and overwhelming it can be when you are giving your all to bring the best possible nutrition to your family and the precious darlings become moody little resisters. It is so tempting to avoid all this food stress and simply serve up what you know your little—and no longer little—ones will eat. Having said that, I also know that with loving tenacity and a few tricks up your sleeve, every growing prince or princess can fall in love with his or her healthy-licious-eating self. Trust me, it can work. It is so satisfying to know that they have come to crave wholesomeness when they search for love, nourishment, and tasty pleasure.

So, what is the secret? How do you transform a fussy, picky, non-vegetable-or healthy-looking food eater into embracing a varied, balanced diet filled with fresh goodness? Stay with me...I'm happy to explain what works for my family and many of the families I have consulted with and coached.

THE PICKY EATER: WHAT WORKS AND WHAT DOES NOT

I had one of those picky eaters in my house. (I am talking joyfully in the past tense, because she is now open to eating a beautifully balanced diet bursting with goodness). When I began introducing new foods, beyond breastmilk, she was very suspicious of everything I gave her and tried very cautiously if she tried at all. She was entirely opposed to any white foods, even in her bottle. She literally drove me crazy. She was an action doll (I wonder where she got her desire for happy-licious movement from?), but she could not have been less interested in food. Hence, I was the mother of a rather thin baby, toddler, and then child. This only strengthened my desire for her to eat. She is my first born and I was worried for her health. I wanted nothing more than to see her thrive.

So, here is what I learnt: The more upset I became about her aversion to new food, the less willing she was to eat anything. She seemed to have an internal sensor that picked right up on my emotions. Sensing my feelings literally locked her mouth shut and nothing would change her mind.

ACTION STEPS TO HELP YOUR LITTLIES FIND THEIR HEALTHY-LICIOUS

1. Keep your cool

Stay as calm as you possibly can be and do not let your emotions get into the way of your child's diet. Instead, learn to trust in your child's innate ability to eat enough to thrive.

Obviously, I completely understand how hard this can be, but it is so important for you both to conquer this. The more relaxed you are, the more relaxed and open your child will be, too.

Know and trust that your child will be absolutely fine. Believe that your child will always eat and drink enough (discounting instances where a child has a condition that does not allow them to align with their natural body wisdom). Some little children seem to live on a diet of deep breaths...but they still have an innate sense of knowing how much they need to eat and drink. If they do not eat at one meal, they will absolutely make up for it at the next. They may snack more, nurse more, or take more bottles. They may ask for additional cheese, crackers, bread, or veggie sticks. One way or another, they will compensate. The more you can release any emotional attachment to the foods your child is choosing to eat or not to eat, the sooner she or he will lose their own inhibitions. Mix your table situation up with a great portion of fun and laughter and you will have soon won your child over.

Did you know that some children feel fear towards new foods? I am 100% certain my daughter did.

2. Trust in repetition

Expose your child to the same nutritious foods continuously and repeatedly.

The more familiar your child becomes with the food, the more daring your little person will become. Try it. I know it is frustrating to cook the same thing over and over again just to have your child push the plate vehemently away, but it feels even more rewarding the first time she or he dives into your delicious creations. Yes, it might take up to 15-20 exposures at your end but, I am here to tell you...it works!!! So, do not give up—keep cooking!!!

3. Variety has power

Expose your child to as many different foods as possible. This will not only allow them to familiarise themselves and their immune systems with a large variety of foods (lowering their risk of allergies), but research shows it will also increase your child's acceptance of foods.

Children who were exposed to several foods seem more willing to actually eat and enjoy their vegetables. Their tastebuds are developing now, so it makes sense to expose them to a mixture of flavours. Innate is their love for sweetness, but if you allow your child to become a little taste explorer, you may spare them a lot of frustrating food battles in later life. If you expose your child to nutritious whole foods early on, it is highly likely that this is what they will go back to. If you dull their tastebuds early in life with too much sugar, salt, and other taste spoilers, you rob them of the amazing experience to nurture themselves with health-boosting whole foods. Obviously, we all do our best and we all make mistakes, so do not beat yourself up over any previous blunders. Every journey is unique, but if you want the easiest, most direct path towards your child wholeheartedly embracing a wholesome diet, then offering the spectrum of flavours, textures, and appearances of whole foods is truly the way to go.

4. Small does not mean insignificant

Always take your child's needs, fears, and food behaviours seriously. Your child's feelings are as real and as valid as yours are. Just as you have your concerns, problems, worries, and fears, so does your child. Your child's feelings are very real for him or her and your child will recognise it if you are meeting his/her needs or whether you are belittling them and their emotions. Just because they are young, does not mean that they do not hold innate knowledge and intuition. They are far more in tune than we think.

This means that you do not try to "outwit" your children by hiding vegetables in their foods. What does this teach them? That vegetables are something that need hiding? No. It is upon you to empower them. They have a right to know what they are eating. Explain to them why you are adding vegetables and why it is important to you and for them. Explain why you are changing from refined grains to whole grains and allow them time while they are transitioning. Mix white rice with brown or mix quinoa with brown rice until their tastes have adapted. Trust me, they will, and quite possibly with a lot of complaining in the beginning, but years later they will not remember this. What they will remember is how Mum's wholesome food tasted, smelled and felt like love.

5. Get Creative

Give your dish a fun, cute and most appetising make-over possible.

I know this might be more time intensive but it is actually really fun, too. And above all, it is incredibly effective. Cut your breads in whimsical shapes or create happy faces with fruit and nut-butters. Serve food that is bright and colourful and offer lots of different textures to your child. Obviously the only creative limit is YOU. Foods that are relatively simple and usually work well include different kinds of spreads in little containers such as hummus, nut-butters, and guacamole. Cut lots of little rainbow sticks out of cucumbers, capsicum, celery, different colours of carrots, sugar snaps or frozen peas, as well as cauliflower and broccoli flowers (aka florets). Empower your children at any age with knowledge of what the different foods can do for their bodies. Make it age-appropriate and fun. Take it from me, any child will love to know that nut-butters make us strong (show strong arms), that avocados make us pretty (make a pretty face), and that carrots can help you grow (show how tall you can reach), etc.

6. Remove any distractions

Turn off electronic distractions or put them aside. Allow your child to discover that mealtimes are about being together as a family and about eating nourishing foods together. It is about exchanging beautiful, positive, and fun experiences. There is no room for books, toys, pacifier, TV, radio, or mum's mobile phone when the family gathers around the table to share a meal. Instead, there is a lot of room for a relaxed atmosphere filled with joyful laughter and happy faces and tummies that feel more satisfied with every wholesome bite.

7. Don't fall into the reward or punishment trap

Resist any temptation to bribe or punish your child with food. Instead, try to stay as relaxed and neutral about the entire food situation. If your child decides not to eat and stays uninterested towards the food put in front of him or her, simply take the plate away after 15 minutes or so. You could say that mealtime is over, and that it is time to play now or get ready for bed, etc., and that we can eat later again. If you bribe your child, rewarding or punishing with food, you may set the grounds for a life-long unhealthy relationship with food. Your child will learn that junk foods are comforting and rewarding and that healthy food is something negative. Arghhh...this is not the path we want to take, and it is definitely not the way to establish a love affair with food and healthy eating. Instead, tell your child what nutrients are in which foods and how those nutrients will help them to become even healthier, smarter, more beautiful, fitter, stronger, etc.

8. Eat together

It goes without saying that our children are like little sponges. They literally soak up all that we do and say (and don't say) like hungry little magnets. Whether you want them to or not, they will mirror what they see. If your children see that you love sitting down with them and eating all the colourful, crunchy, healthy-licious whole foods yourself, they will be much more likely to do so, too. If you show them all the pleasure you get out of eating such wonderfully nurturing meals, they will be much more likely to do so, too. If you are commenting on how totally amazing those foods make you feel, they are much more likely to embrace nutritious foods as wholesome nourishment for body, mind and soul.

Unfortunately, I still see so many parents eating at different times to their children and also eating different foods. How very confusing is such behaviour for those little open minds and eyes? What message does this send for their own isolated relationship with food? Again, it is not about making everything perfect, it is about creating an atmosphere of enjoyed togetherness, of warm caring and delightful happiness.

9. Get your child cooking with you

This one is the most fun for both of you. Allow her or him to be involved somewhere along the long line of producing food onto the table. Take your child shopping with you and empower them by letting them decide upon one of the different kinds of fruits, vegetables, nuts, whole grains or seeds to buy. Pick fresh produce with them from the garden. Let them help you wash and prepare the foods—obviously keeping the work age appropriate (knives do not belong in the hands of toddlers). You will be truly surprised by how much your child actually enjoys being a part of this wholesome cooking creation. You will be astonished by their willingness to fall in love with their healthy creations.

10. Be Hands-On

Allow your child to explore their foods with their hands. Hands-on littlies become teens who know their way around the kitchen—and hopefully do not have to eat with their hands anymore. The early exploration period sets the stage for them to accept and love whole foods, know what food combinations they love and how to be self-sufficient. Yes, putting up with a messy child and kitchen can be so worth it. This hands-on stuff translates into capable adults.

THE SAD FACTS

It is not only our waistlines that are growing, but our children's bellies are, too. This isn't "baby fat is cute," this is "childhood obesity rates that have never been higher" scary. We need to start talking about this and we need to start taking this seriously. We need to address this. NOW!!!

We cannot ignore any longer the fact that our children have become sedentary, that they struggle to run, jump, and explore in the ways that characterize a happy childhood. They will not outgrow being immobile and sluggish. Children sitting and overeating their way through their developmental years are at an increased risk of disease and early death. They are not chubby because they are children. They are obese because they are neglected. So, what is going on? Quite simply, we have allowed our own poor health choices to trickle down to our children. We have set them up for an even bigger challenge than we face, creating unnecessary challenges to their own healthy-licious journey. This is unfair because it is not their fault. They too are victims of growing portion sizes, too much sugar in our foods, way too much packaged, pre-cooked and processed foods, misleading marketing, and to top it off, commercials with all the wrong messages. They too are victims of a society that is increasingly moving less, but eating more. Computer games have never been more addictive and regulating our children around screen time never felt harder. But it is not all bad. The good news is there is always a way out...because we always have a choice in life to change, to turn things around and even to start all over. It is time to do so, and I have plenty of ideas on how to change gears and move in the right direction.

What to do?

This is the wake-up call. This is the time to jump back into action and wake up from this insane body-disconnectedness we have fallen into.

It is not about being skinny or perfect. It is about being the healthiest, most vibrant, happiest version of yourself. It starts at any age, and it starts with you.

Are you ready to teach your sons and daughters how good it feels to embark on a happy relationship with oneself? To nurture your body instead of stuffing it? We have learnt that stuffing our body with food just stuffs the emotions down deeper, ignoring that we can deal with life's challenges and disappointments. It is like stuffing your body into silence—its voice muffled by fat, distracted by disease, silenced by resistance to change. Are you open to listen again to all the subtle messages of your body instead of overstepping boundaries of portion sizes and making sometimes-foods the source of primary fuel? The more you learn to respect, accept and love your body, the more you will demonstrate such loving behaviour to your offspring. You are their biggest role model.

TAKE LITTLE BABY STEPS CONTINUOUSLY

1. Empower your children with knowledge and/or find support who will do so with or for you. I know too well that from a certain age, everything you say or do is pretty uncool, so it might be more effective enlisting a mentor your child admires to be your partner in sending these important messages to your son or daughter.

2. Get them engaged and interested in healthy cooking, gardening, shopping, healthy eating workshops, etc. Cooking together has no age expiry date. Creating something healthy-licious together can be a truly beautiful bonding experience. Go to a bookstore together and choose together a cookbook that features lots of new wholesome recipes you would both like to try.

3. Be active together. Leave the car more often at home and take instead your bikes or simply enjoy the flowing strength of your beautiful legs. Enrol in a yoga or gym class together or try a YouTube video at home. Have some fun together. Show your child how wonderful it feels to move all the energy they hold in their beautiful bodies. Allow them to notice how exercise quiets the mind, takes away the worry, and lifts their spirit. Allow them to tune back into their physical selves instead of becoming numb towards their bodies. I think the best Christmas presents I could have ever given my daughters one year were a pair of skates each, two pairs of boxing gear and two Fit-bits. They work...they keep my girls up and about, moving around and they are even on trend with their hip accessories (very important, of course, for young teenagers!).

4. Explore the concept of the different forms of hunger with your children. Choose to eat mindfully together, being aware not to fall into any of those horrible hunger traps. It can be quite fun to speak this secret hunger language together with your kids. I will ask for example: "which hunger do you think is talking now?" And they will stop for a moment and then say, "thirst hunger...oops, got confused." Then, I will do the same—it really is kind of fun, especially when we have friends over who think we are complete nutters (which of course we are!!!).

5. Support and guide them to eat more vegetables and less junk. The more you make whole foods accessible as the main source of food in your home, the more they will choose such foods for nourishment. Load your fridge with fresh, healthy-licious fruits and vegetables in all the beautiful colours of the rainbow. Stock your pantry with whole grains, beans, nuts, seeds and seaweed.

6. Be mindful of not simply taking foods out of your children's diet, but instead to lovingly replace them with more nutritious alternatives. If your child is used to drinking a lot of juice or soft drinks, replace with sparkling water with a few spritzers of fruit juice to add some yummy flavour. If your child is

used to snacking on potato crisps in the afternoon, make a big batch of crispy, spicy (or not so spicy) roasted chickpeas. Try serving seaweed or nuts and seeds over freshly cut-up fruits for some added flavour, crunch and yumminess. If your child would usually start the day on a big load of sugary cereals, satisfy their overstimulated tastebuds with spices like cinnamon, nutmeg, cardamom, etc., or less aggressive forms of sweeteners in lower amounts, so they can gently adjust.

7. Safeguard your child's sleep. Share with them how sleeping is a form of self-nurture, too and, if age appropriate, explain all the effects not sleeping enough has on their precious bodies.

8. Encourage your child to drink more water. Equip him or her with the gorgeous, fun drink bottles. Come up with water drinking competitions where everyone reports back every evening as to how many bottles of water they drank during the day. The winner of one week gets a small prize such as a gold coin or a pretty lip-balm. The winner of the month gets extra quality time with mum. I love this game because it ticks all the boxes—it not only increases my child's desire to drink more, it also makes me drink more. (Hey, I have a competitive streak inside of me, too... I want that pretty lip-balm in my pocket, plus I get to spend more quality time with my awesome princesses at the end of every month. Win-win-win!)

WHAT ABOUT OLDER CHILDREN AND TEENAGERS?

I am very deeply concerned for all those teenagers out there. They are even more confused than we are. They are confronted with so many different ideas, emotions and information. They are only just starting to work out who they truly are, something both exciting and frightening. They have the overwhelming desire to fit in with the big crowd, while also wanting their own identity, to be special, to shine, and to stand out—but only in admirable ways. They are bombarded by media advertising and are so vulnerable to the subtle innuendo about physical perfection. Social media holds overwhelming power over our children. In a world where daily selfies are normal, they are exposed to constant comparison with what they perceive as perfect. I am so glad I am not a teenager in this time. I do not think I would have responded well to the pressure to be perfect. The unhealthy ways children are programmed to relate to themselves is scary and the consequences are devastating. There has never been a generation that has struggled more from eating disorders, body dissatisfaction, and body-mind disconnection. The truth of healthy eating and being physically active has never been more misunderstood.

Action Steps to empower your teens toward radiant health

1. ALWAYS focus on promoting well-being and health rather than body shape, size, or weight. Ask them how certain foods make them feel, and how they affect their skin, hair, and nails. Are there any foods that make them feel more calm, or more focused? What foods do they notice that increase fear, anxiety, or nervousness? Do certain foods make them feel full and do some give them a longer lasting full feeling than others? Are there foods that make them moody, angry, or irritated? Are there foods that make your child feel beautiful, clever, creative, or inspired?

2. Do not be afraid to get professional help if you feel overwhelmed and know your child is struggling with nourishing his or her body the healthy way. The sooner you take action, the easier it will be for your teen to find new, healthful ways.

   The positive side of the obesity coin is: with our children's waistlines on the rise, so are more and more highly qualified professionals to help you deal with any form of food struggles.

How to know which support is right for you and your teen? Learn the difference:

Dieticians

Dietitians provide expert advice on nutrition and will prescribe diet plans for their clients to follow. They are also qualified to prescribe dietary treatments for clients who present with diabetes, food intolerances, cardiovascular disease, gastrointestinal issues, underweight, eating disorders, overweight and obesity.

Nutritionists

Nutritionists provide advice in regards to food choices. They work with their clients to help them optimise their health and well-being through diet. They generally do not work with clients who suffer from severe medical issues and their services are nutrition related only.

Nutrition Coach

Nutrition Coaches guide, support, and empower their clients to replace old behaviours with new ones, develop strategies that will help them reach their goals, and motivate them to keep going when things become too difficult for them. These can be nutrition related, but can also include aspects of the client's overall holistic health and well-being.

3. Support your child in learning and understanding what a healthy body looks like. Empower your teen with the bitter truth around airbrushed pictures in glossy magazines, how posing from certain angles can change the entire look from "perfect Instagram idol" to normal-has-thighs-and-a-belly-too look.

ADDITIONAL ACTION STEPS TO ENCOURAGE POSITIVE BODY IMAGE:

1. Help your teen to appreciate their body by helping them to name all the things their body does for them on a daily basis.

2. Regularly tell your teen things you love about them that has nothing to do with how they look or their body shape and size.

3. Ensure your teen moves their body regularly in ways they enjoy to feel strong, fit, and good in their beautiful skin—not for weight loss reasons.

4. Help your teen to focus on qualities they value more than physical looks. (Do they love their friends for their looks or because they are kind, fun, creative, caring, supportive, loyal, a good listener, etc.?) Share frequently with them what you value and look for in a friend.

5. Support your teen to focus on her own beautiful self instead of falling into the negative trap of comparison.

6. Help your child to replace negative self-talk with the positive truth.

Let's Get Cooking

I do not claim to be a particularly good cook, or present myself as an expert on the subject, I just happen to really love eating—but not just any kind of food, of course. I love to nurture my body, soul, and mind with foods that make me feel amazing and bring my very best out in me.

My recipes feature dishes, meals, and drinks that are quick and easy for me to make and fit beautifully into my busy life. Some I have recreated from childhood memories and others I may have tasted in restaurants. Some recipes may have been inspired by or felt a stroke of social media and inspiration that I have simply re-created in a dish in a Healthy-licious way and others I have dreamt up from good old experimentation. One thing is certain: my recipes are all full of wholesome, health-boosting, beautifying, feel-good ingredients. Consider reading them for a general guideline and then adapt to your tastes, circumstances, and needs. We are all so different when it comes to our likes and dislikes, budget, environment and circumstances in general. It is these differences which make creating dishes so special and exciting for us home cooks.

So let your creative cooking spirits flow, do it with love for yourself and those you cook for, and above all—ENJOY.

RECIPES

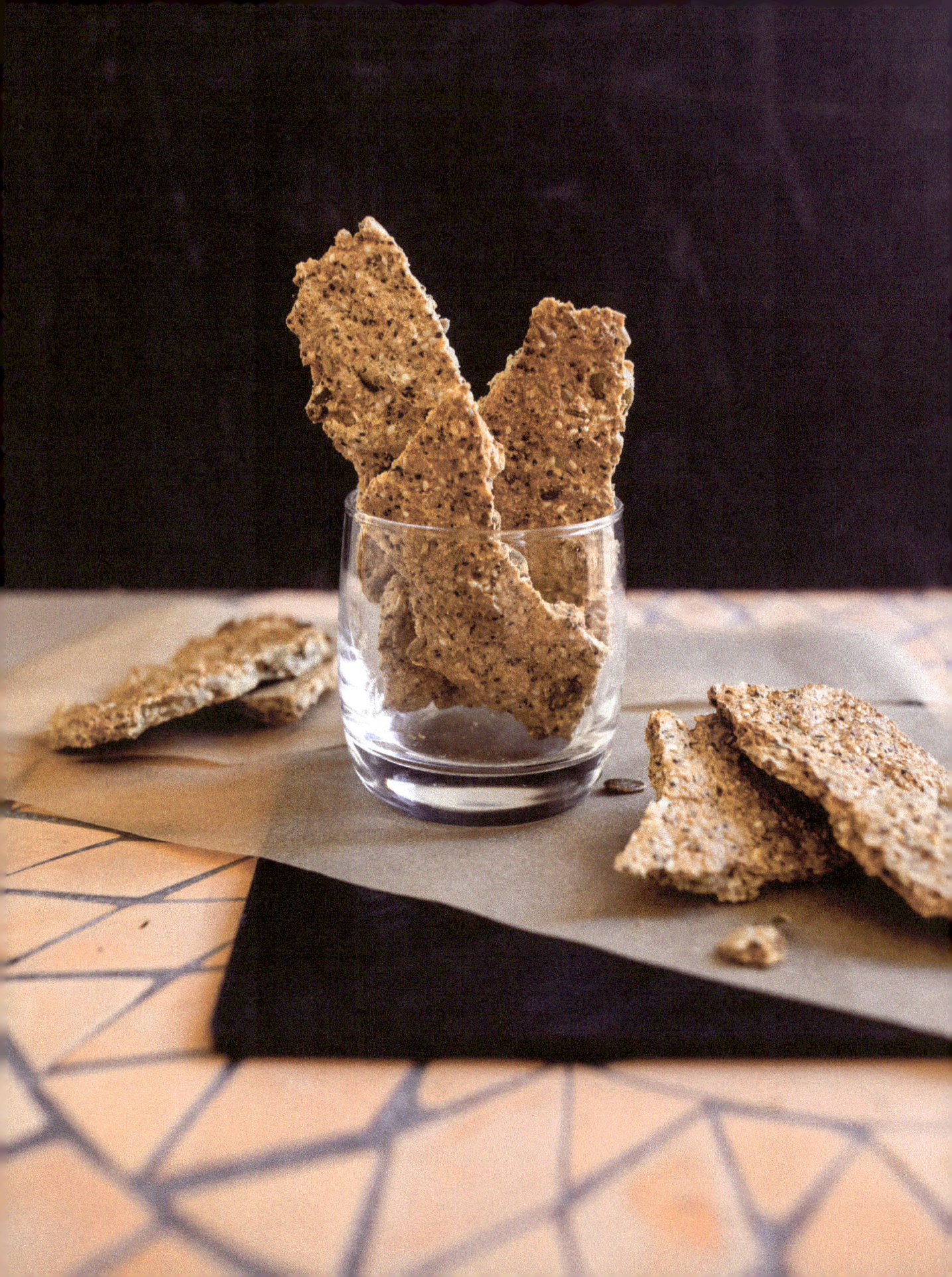

ALL-TOO-EASY SEEDED CRISP BREADS

MAKES: 12 CRISPBREADS (depending on how you slice them)

INGREDIENTS:

- 1 cup of raw almonds
- ½ cup of rolled oats or quinoa flakes
- ½ tsp of gluten-free baking powder (make your own: ½ tsp of bicarbonate of soda, 1 tsp of cream of tartar and 1 cup of gluten-free flour. I like to use brown rice and mill it into flour. Store leftovers in an airtight container)
- ½ tsp of good-quality salt (I love to use herbal salt for this one, Herbamare is a good one)
- ½ cup of mixed seeds (sunflower and pepita)
- 3 TBSP of chia seeds
- 6 TBSP of water
- ¼ cup of sesame seeds
- 2 TBSP of nutritional yeast flakes
- Optional: 2 eggs
- 2 TBSP of extra virgin olive oil

METHOD:

1. Preheat your oven to 150°C and line your baking tray with baking paper.
2. In a small bowl, mix your chia seeds with 6–7 TBSP of water. Stir frequently and set aside until a glutinous gel forms.
3. In your food processor, process your almonds into a fine almond meal and combine with oats or quinoa flakes, baking powder, salt, all your seeds and nutritional yeast flakes. Make sure your sunflower and pepita seeds are only chopped, not totally ground.
4. Add your wet ingredients (chia seed mixture, olive oil and eggs if using) and mix until well combined.
5. Spread your dough onto the prepared tray (with baking paper) as thinly as possible and bake for 20–30 minutes or until your crispbreads are golden brown and smell totally irresistible.

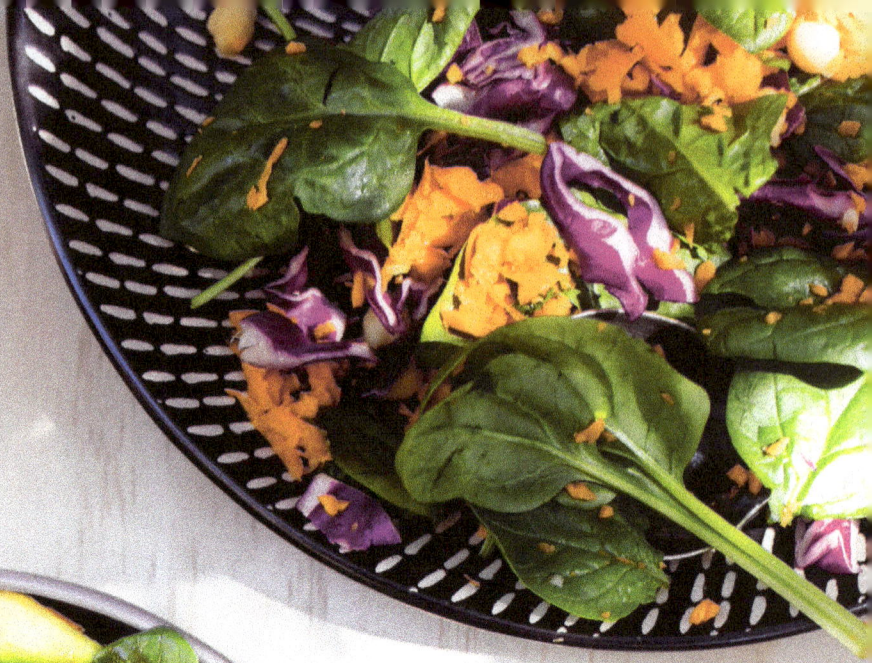

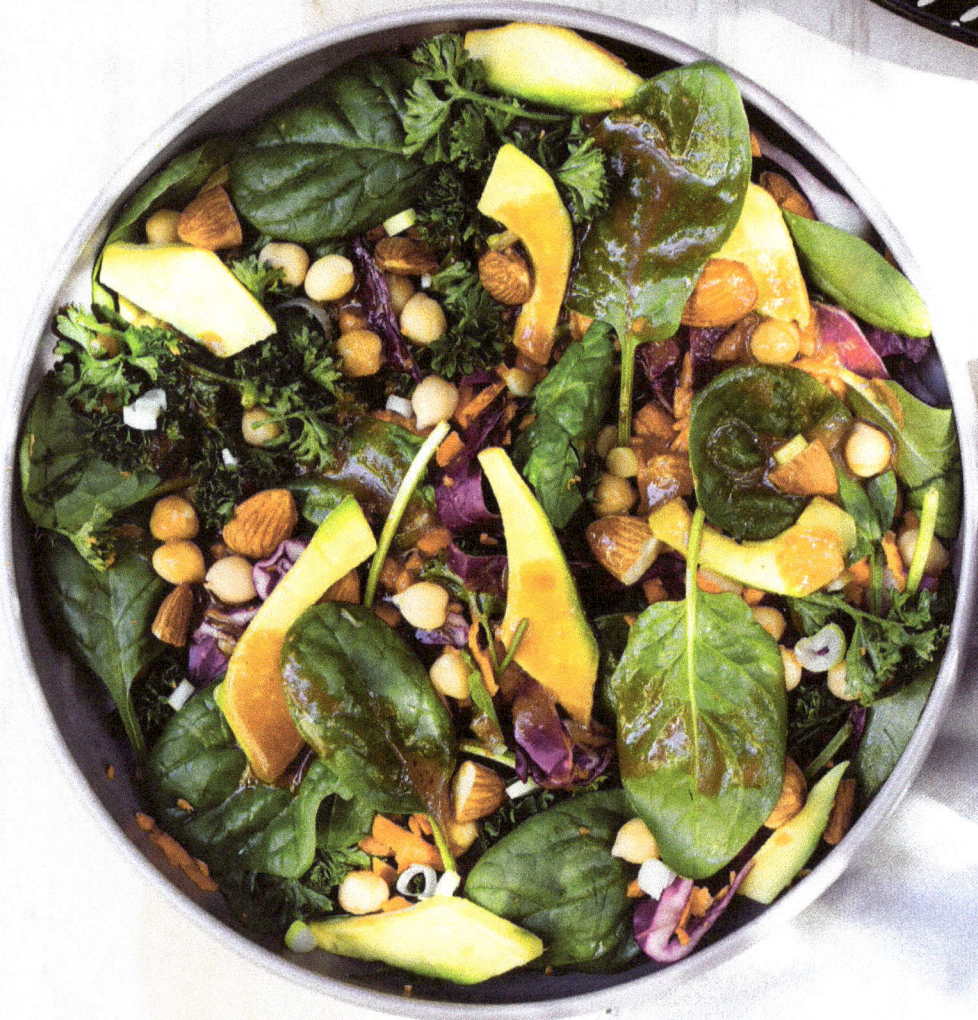

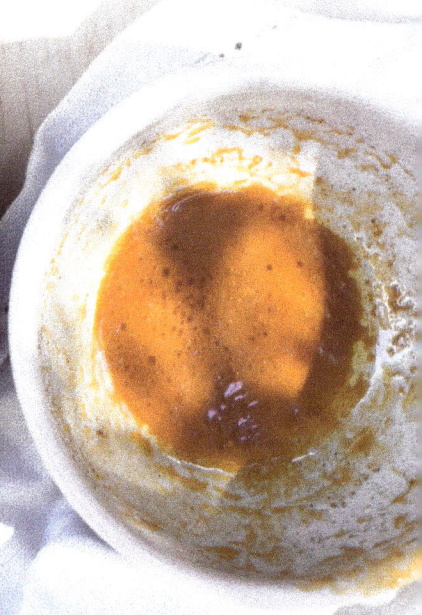

ANTI-AGEING CARROT SALAD

MAKES: 4 BOWLS

SALAD:

- 8 medium carrots, grated or 4 cups grated
- ¼ head of purple cabbage, thinly shredded
- 3–4 cups of fresh spinach leaves
- 1 tin of chickpeas, thoroughly rinsed and drained
- 1 small avocado, diced or sliced into thin wedges
- ¼ cup of raw almonds; optional: roast almonds for 2–3 minutes without using any oil
- 1 cup of parsley, chopped

DRESSING:

- 1.5 tsp of miso paste
- 3 TBSP of tahini
- 3 TBSP of lemon juice
- 1 TBSP of apple cider vinegar
- 1 garlic, crushed
- 1 TBSP of freshly grated ginger
- Good-quality salt and black pepper to taste
- 1–2 spring onion, thinly sliced

METHOD:

1. In a small bowl, whisk together your ingredients for the dressing. Add 2 TBSP of water if consistency of dressing is too thick. Set dressing aside.
2. In a larger bowl or salad dish, add your spinach leaves, shredded cabbage, grated carrots, chickpeas, avocado and sprinkle with parsley. If using roasted almonds, briefly roast them in a small pan over medium heat for 2–3 minutes without using any oil. Toss or stir them frequently to avoid burning. Top your salad mixture with raw or roasted nuts.
3. Drizzle your dressing over your salad.

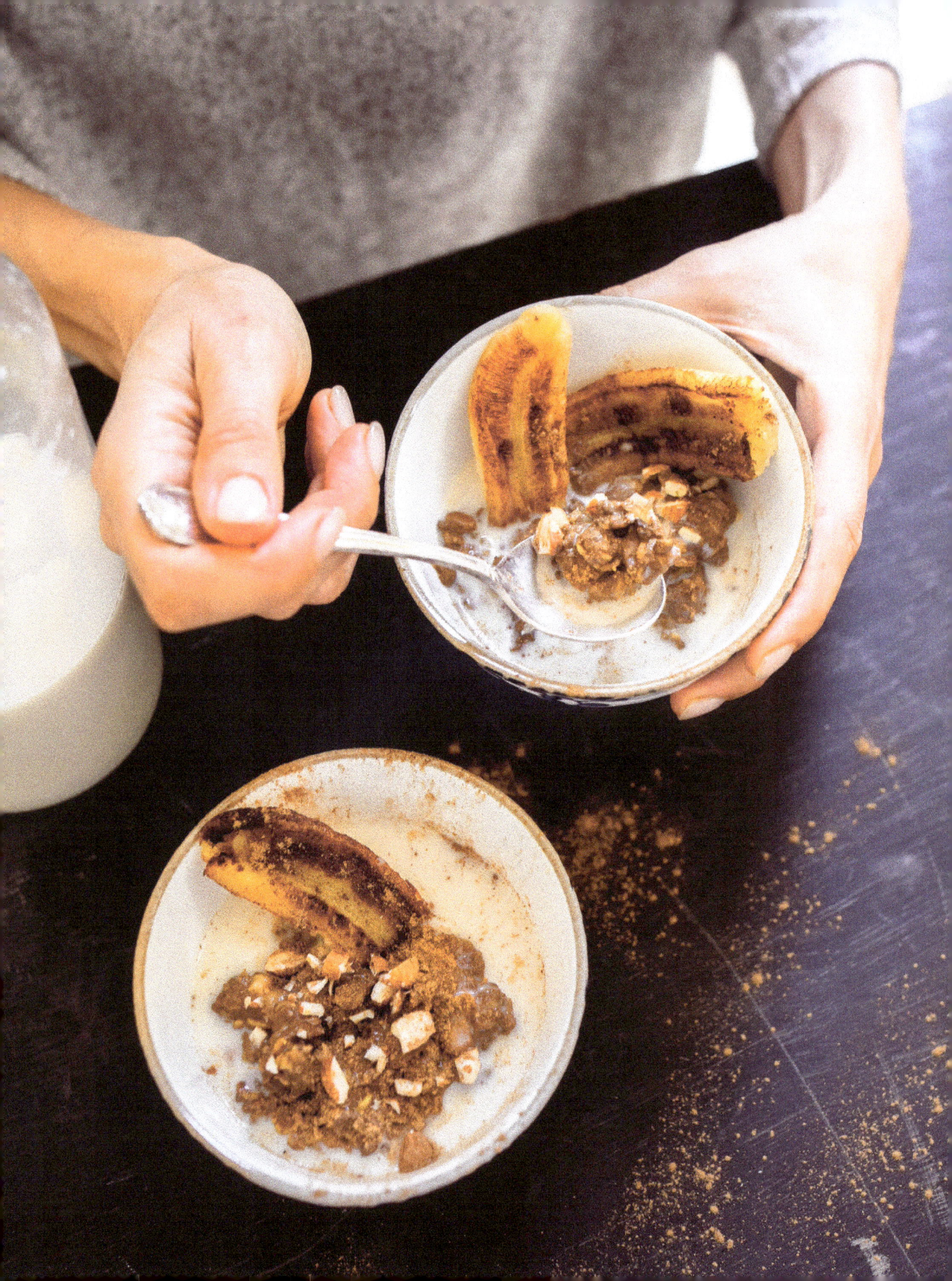

BEAUTIFYING CHAI CHOCOLATE PORRIDGE

MAKES: 2 BOWLS

INGREDIENTS:

- 1 cup of rolled or steel-cut oats
- At least 2 cups of unsweetened almond milk (I like my porridge very creamy, so I like adding more milk)
- 1–2 TBSP of raw cacao powder
- 1 tsp of turmeric, ground
- 1 tsp of pure vanilla bean, ground
- ½ tsp of cinnamon
- Pinch of clove, ground (optional, but clove has insanely high antioxidant properties, more than most other foods)
- Pinch of nutmeg, ground
- ¼ tsp of ginger, ground or small piece of fresh ginger, grated
- Pinch of black pepper, ground
- 1–2 tsp of rice malt syrup
- 2 small ripe bananas
- 2 TBSP of black chia seeds

Optional: 2 tsp of maca powder
Optional: 2 scoops of collagen powder, preferably unsweetened
Mixed berries
Optional: sprinkle with handful of nuts of your choice such as almonds, walnuts and Brazil nuts

METHOD:

1. In a small saucepan, combine your oats, milk, spices and rice malt syrup, and simmer on low heat with closed lid, stirring frequently until most the milk has been absorbed by the oats. Consistency should be creamy, not too dense, so you can still mix with the rest of the ingredients. Depending on your stove, this takes 5–8 minutes.
2. Meanwhile, mash your bananas and put each mashed banana into one porridge bowl.
3. Add 1 TBSP of chia seeds to each of the bowls filled with the mashed banana, mix well and then set aside.
4. Remove your porridge from the heat and pour into your prepared bowls. Add your maca and collagen powder, if using, and combine well with your mashed banana–chia seed mixture.
5. Add your choice of berries and stir through lightly.
6. Sprinkle with your favourite nuts.

AVO-LICIOUS BERRY POPSICLES

MAKES: 12 POPSICLES

INGREDIENTS:

- 3 cups frozen or fresh berries (any kind or mixed is delicious)
- 1 ripe banana
- 1 ripe avocado
- 1 tsp of pure ground vanilla bean
- 2 cups almond milk, unsweetened
- 2 TBSP of chia seeds

METHOD:

1. In a small bowl, mix your chia seeds into your almond milk. Stir and then let it sit to thicken and form a glutinous gel for 10–15 minutes.
2. In the meantime, place all your fruit and spice into your blender, add your almond milk–chia seed mixture and avocado, and mix until well combined.
3. Pour your berry-licious nice-cream mixture into your popsicle moulds and freeze for 4–6 hours.

BERRY-LICIOUS BREAKFAST CRUMBLE

MAKES: 4 PORTIONS

INGREDIENTS:

- 1 cup of frozen blueberries
- 1 cup of frozen raspberries
- 1 cup of frozen strawberries
- (or 3 cups of mixed berries)
- 1 cup of rolled oats
- ¼ cup of sunflower seeds
- ¼ cup of desiccated coconut, unsweetened
- 2 TBSP of walnuts, roughly chopped
- 2 TBSP of almond, roughly chopped
- 1 tsp of ground cinnamon, unsweetened
- 1 tsp of pure vanilla bean, ground
- Pinch of good-quality salt
- 1–2 TBSP of rice malt syrup
- 2 TBSP of liquid coconut oil

METHOD:

1. Line your baking dish with baking paper and pre-heat the oven to 160°C or lightly grease each ramekin with oil.
2. Add your frozen berries to your prepared dish(es) and set aside.
3. Place your oats, sunflower seeds, desiccated coconut and nuts in a large mixing bowl and combine well.
4. In a small pot, heat your coconut oil, rice malt syrup, salt and spices, and heat until mixture liquifies. Stir to combine well.
5. Remove from the heat and pour coconut oil mixture over your oat and seed mixture until it is well coated.
6. Pour your crumble mixture over your prepared baking dish or ramekins filled with berries.
7. Bake in the oven for 30–35 minutes or until your crumble is golden brown and smells irresistible.

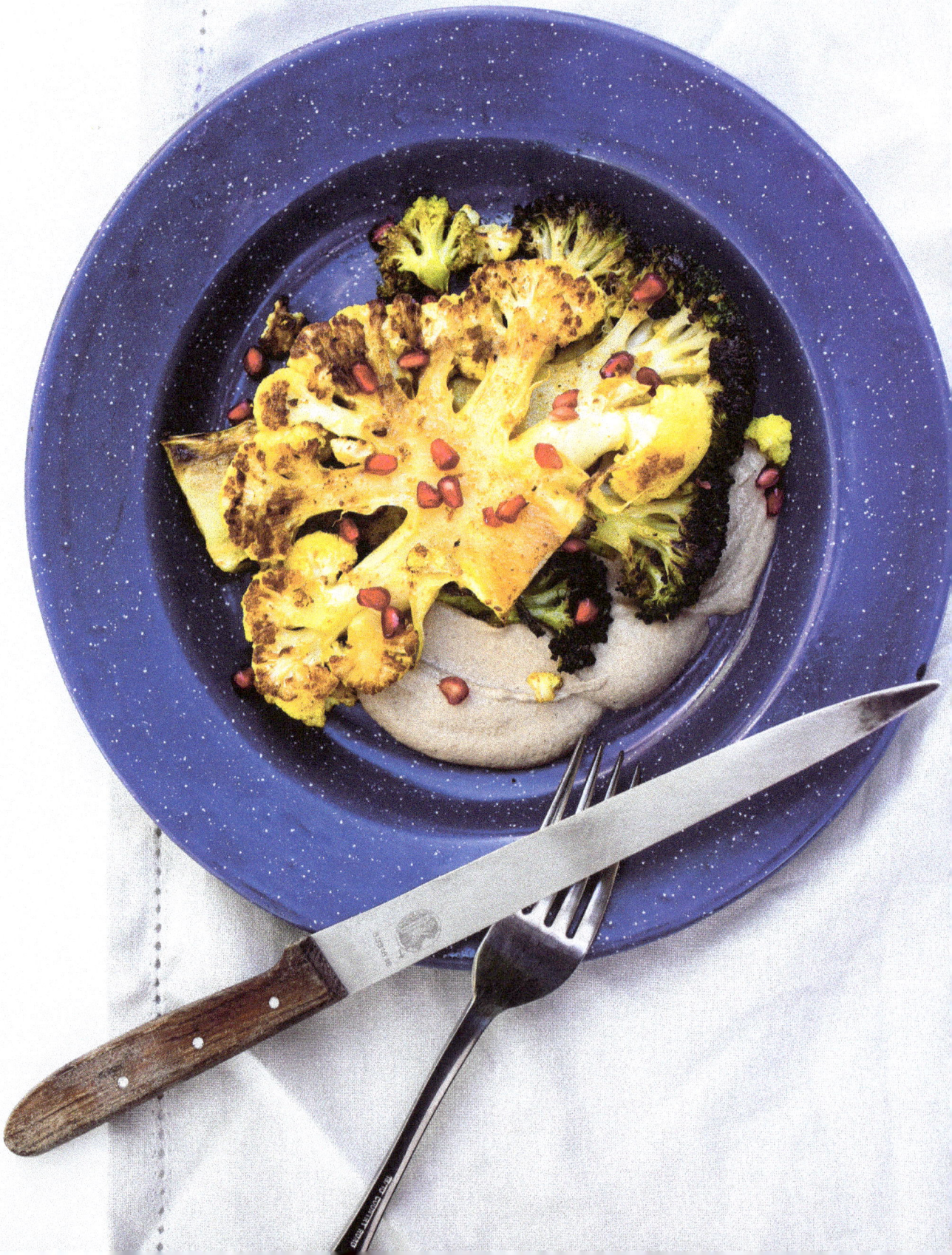

BROCCOLI AND CAULIFLOWER STEAKS WITH LEMON TAHINI DRESSING

MAKES: 4 PORTIONS

FOR THE BROCCOLI AND CAULIFLOWER STEAKS:

- 1 medium to large head of cauliflower, sliced lengthwise into 4 x 1-cm-thick slices or steaks
- 1 medium to large head of broccoli, sliced lengthwise into 4 x 1-cm-thick slices or steaks
- ½ cup of extra virgin olive oil
- 1 tsp of ground turmeric
- 1 tsp of ground cumin
- ¼ tsp of ground chilli
- Salt and black pepper, cracked to taste
- ½ cup of almonds, roughly chopped

FOR THE LEMON TAHINI DRESSING:

- ¼ cup of water, filtered
- ½ cup of tahini, unhulled
- ¼ cup of lemon juice, freshly squeezed
- ¼ cup of apple cider vinegar, raw with mother
- 1 garlic, crushed
- 1 TBSP of grated ginger
- Good-quality salt and black pepper to taste
- 1 tsp of rice malt syrup

Optional: Sprinkle with ½ cup of pomegranate seeds

METHOD:

1. Cut your broccoli and cauliflower according to directions.
2. In a smaller bowl, mix together your oil and spices.
3. Brush both sides of your broccoli and cauliflower steaks generously with your oil mixture.
4. Heat a large frying pan and put first 4 steaks (2 cauliflower-, 2 broccoli-steaks) and fry each side for about 5 minutes or until tops are golden and crispy and vegetables cooked. Steaks turn golden and crispy.
5. In the meantime, using another smaller bowl, mix together your lemon tahini dressing until smooth and creamy.
6. Once your first batch of broccoli and cauliflower steaks is cooked, set them aside and repeat the cooking process with second batch.
7. To assemble your dish, spoon lemon tahini dressing over your roasted broccoli and cauliflower steaks and sprinkle with pomegranate seeds, if using.

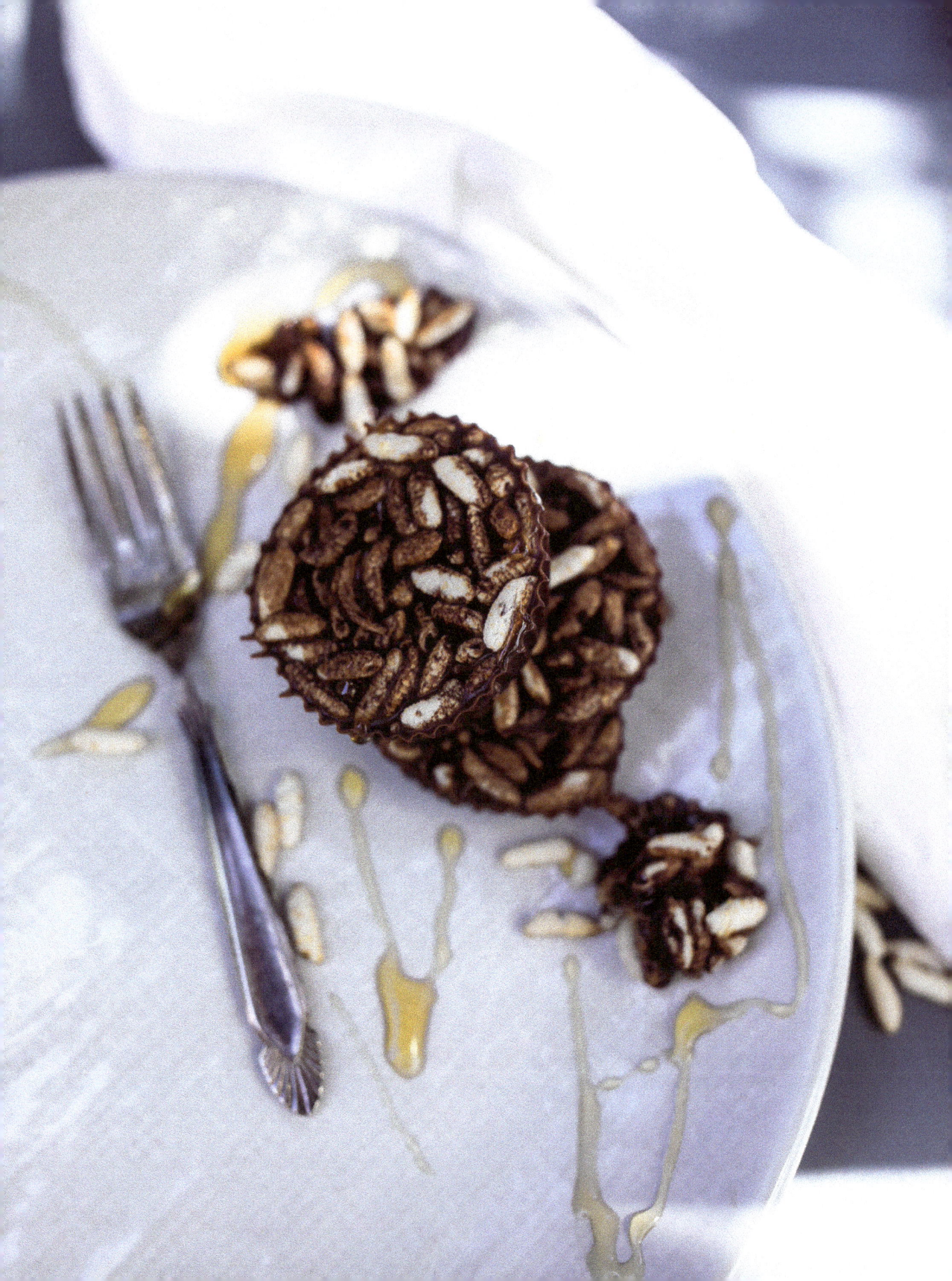

CHILLI CHOCOLATE RICE PUFFS

MAKES 12 SQUARES OR CLUSTERS

INGREDIENTS:

- ½ cup of virgin coconut oil
- ¼ cup of raw cocoa powder
- ¼ cup of rice malt syrup
- Pinch of chilli powder, for more of a punch use ¼ tsp of chilli powder
- Pinch of sea salt
- 1 cup of brown rice pops, unsweetened

METHOD:

1. Line a freezer-proof dish with baking paper and fill the base with your rice pops; alternatively use little paper moulds and fill the base of each with rice pops.
2. In a small pot, melt the coconut oil.
3. Stir in cocoa powder, rice malt syrup, spice and salt.
4. Pour your chocolate mixture over your rice pops, making sure you cover ever pop with some chocolate.
5. Place your baking dish or moulds into the freezer for 1 hour.
6. If using a baking dish, cut your Chilli Chocolate Rice Puffs into 12 squares with a wet knife. Store your Chilli Chocolate Rice Puffs in the freezer.

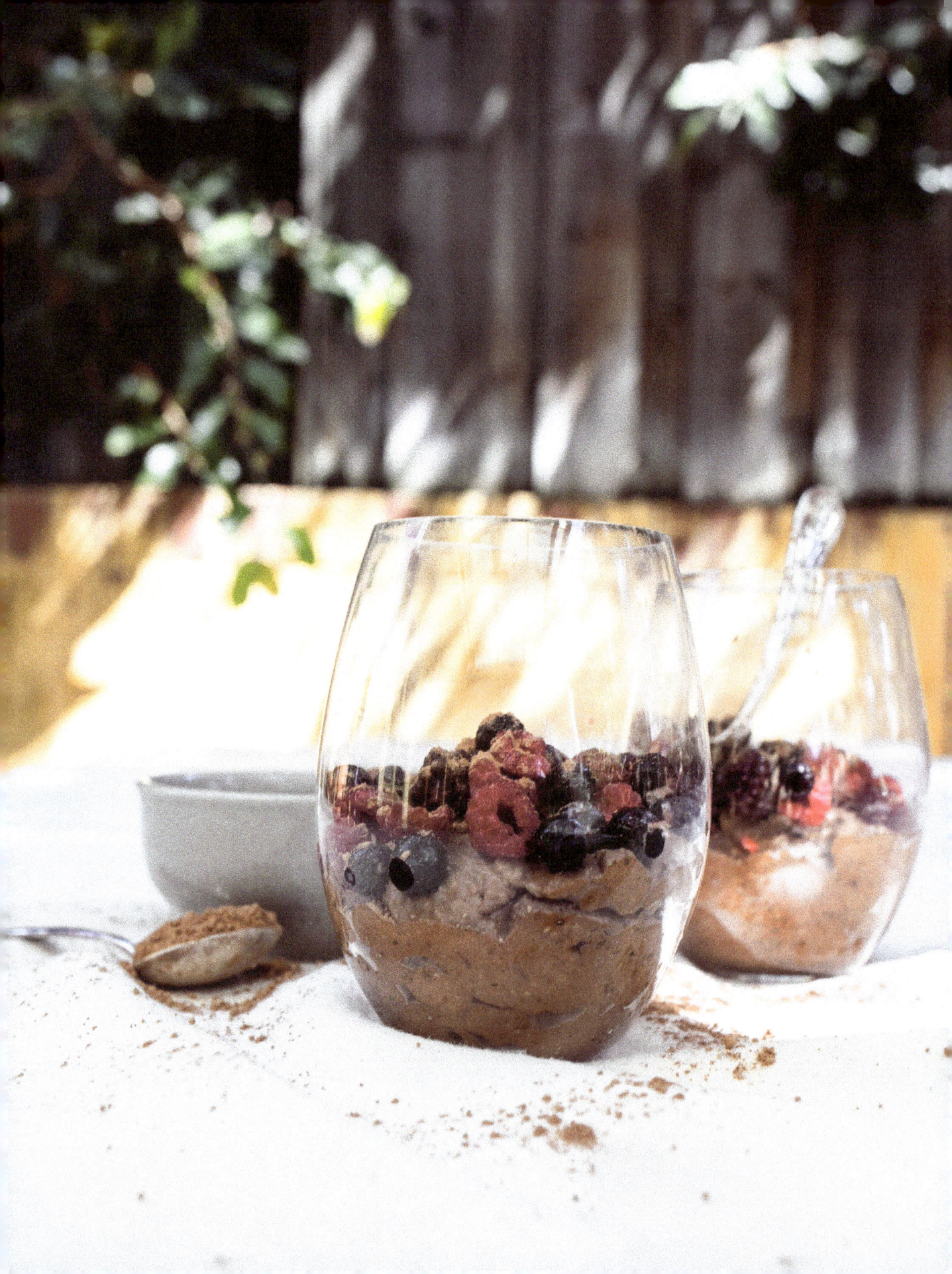

CHOCO-LICIOUS BEAUTY BOWL

MAKES: 2 SERVINGS

INGREDIENTS:

- 2 large ripe bananas, sliced and frozen
- 1–2 TBSP of rice malt syrup (for me even 1 tsp is enough, but you might prefer it sweeter)
- 1 cup of coconut cream, full-fat, unsweetened
- ¼ cup of raw cacao powder
- 1 tsp of pure ground vanilla bean
- ½ tsp of cinnamon
- 2 TBSP of chia seeds

Optional: 1 TBSP of maca powder

METHOD:

1. Place all your ingredients into your high-speed blender and mix until well combined and the texture is creamy smooth.
2. Top with fresh or frozen berries and a small handful of pumpkin seeds!

CRUNCHY-LICIOUS CHOCOLATE BARK

MAKES: 12 SERVINGS

INGREDIENTS:

- 1 cup of coconut oil, melted
- 1 cup of raw cacao powder, unsweetened
- 1 cup of rice malt syrup
- 4 TBSP of hulled or unhulled tahini
- 1 tsp of pure unsweetened vanilla bean, ground
- 1 tsp of cinnamon (optional)
- 1 cup of raw or dry roasted almond, chopped
- 1 cup of mixed seeds (pepita, sunflower and chia)
- 1 cup of frozen mixed berries
- Pinch of good-quality coarse salt to sprinkle on top

METHOD:

1. Line your baking tray with paper and set aside.
2. Mix your coconut oil, cacao powder, rice malt syrup, tahini and spices until well combined.
3. Carefully mix in the nuts, seeds and frozen berries.
4. Pour mixture into your tray and sprinkle with sea salt.
5. Put in freezer for 20 minutes or until completely set. Break your bark into bite-sized pieces and enjoy. Store leftovers in an airtight container in the freezer!

DAL FOR RADIANT BEAUTY

MAKES: 4 SERVINGS

INGREDIENTS:

- 1 TBSP of olive oil
- 1 brown onion, chopped
- 1 small knob of fresh ginger, finely chopped or grated
- 1 TBSP of yellow mustard seeds
- 1 TBSP of cumin seeds
- 1 TBSP of turmeric, ground
- 1 TBSP of Garam Masala
- 1 cup of red lentils (rinsed and drained)
- 3–4 cups of water
- 1/2 head of large cauliflower, cut into florets
- 1 small head of broccoli, cut into florets
- 1 red capsicum, cubed
- 3–5 TBSP of tomato passata
- Good-quality salt and black pepper to taste

METHOD:

1. Heat olive oil over medium heat in a large pan, wok or pot. Add chopped onion, ginger and spices. Sauté until onion is translucent. Stir frequently to prevent spices from burning.
2. Add red lentils and sauté for another 1–2 minutes.
3. Add water tomato passata, salt, pepper and bring to boil.
4. Simmer for about 30 minutes. Add your veggies and additional water if needed. Continue to simmer for another 30 minutes or until all your veggies are cooked and the Dal has a creamy consistency.
5. Enjoy with quinoa, millet, brown or cauliflower rice.

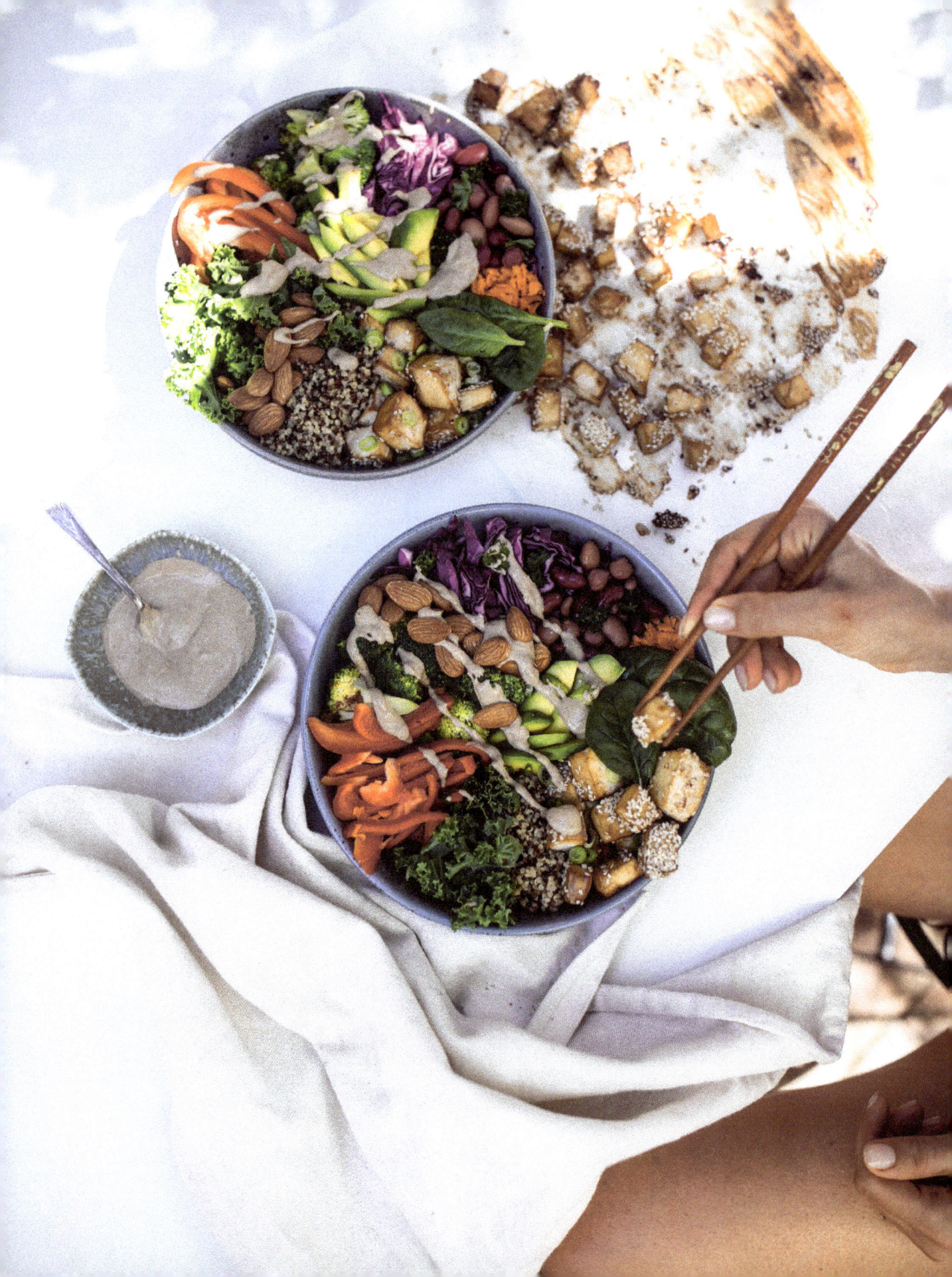

GODDESS BUDDHA BOWL

MAKES: 2 SERVINGS

INGREDIENTS:

BUDDHA BOWL:

- ½ cup of uncooked quinoa, rinsed and drained (I really like tri-coloured quinoa, but any is great)
- ¾ cup of good-quality vegetable broth
- 225 g of firm tofu, drained
- ¼ cup of salt-reduced tamari sauce
- ¼ cup of raw apple cider vinegar
- ¼ cup of raw sesame seeds
- ¼ head of large to medium-sized broccoli, cut into florets
- 1 TBSP of extra virgin olive oil
- Good-quality salt and black pepper to taste
- 1 cup of spinach leaves
- 1 cup of kale leaves
- ¼ head of red cabbage, thinly sliced
- 1 red capsicum, thinly sliced
- ¼ cup of shredded carrot (about 1 medium carrot)
- 1 avocado, thinly sliced
- 1 tin of organic mixed beans, thoroughly rinsed and drained
- 1 spring onion, thinly sliced
- ½ cup of fresh parsley
- ½ cup of almonds, raw or slightly roasted

DRESSING:

- ¼ cup of unhulled tahini
- 2 TBSP of lemon juice
- 1 TBSP of apple cider vinegar
- 1 garlic, crushed
- 1 TBSP of grated ginger
- Optional: rice malt syrup to taste
- Good-quality salt and black pepper to taste
- ¼ cup of warm water

METHOD:

1. Cook your quinoa in ¾ cup of good-quality vegetable broth for about 30–35 minutes over low to medium heat.
2. Prepare a baking tray with baking paper and pre-heat the oven to 180°C.
3. In the meantime, drain your tofu and cut into cubes. In a small bowl, whisk together your salt-reduced tamari sauce and apple cider vinegar. Marinade your tofu in the sauce. Put your marinated tofu onto the prepped baking dish and sprinkle generously with sesame seeds. Put into the oven and roast for 30–35 minutes or until golden brown and crispy.
4. Cut your broccoli into little florets, drizzle with oil, sprinkle with salt and pepper and sauté in your wok or pan for 10–15 minutes or until cooked but still crunchy.
5. Meanwhile, prep all your other vegetables: grate your carrot, shred your cabbage, slice your capsicum, spring onion and avocado, wash and destem your kale leaves and rip into smaller pieces, wash your spinach leaves. Chop your parsley and almonds.
6. Rinse and drain your mixed beans and set aside.
7. To prepare your sauce, add all of your ingredients and mix well; add salt, pepper and possibly rice malt syrup to taste and set aside.
8. To assemble, start making a bed of spinach and kale leaves, add your cooked quinoa, then add the different coloured vegetables, avocado, mixed beans, roasted tofu cubes and cooked broccoli. Top with your fresh herbs, raw chopped nuts and then drizzle tahini dressing on top.

HERB AND MACADAMIA-CRUSTED SALMON

MAKES: 4 SERVINGS

INGREDIENTS:

- 1–1.5 cups of macadamia nuts, chopped
- ¼ cup of parsley, chopped
- ¼ cup of basil leaves, chopped
- 2 TBSP of chives, chopped
- 1 garlic clove, crushed
- 2 TBSP of lemon juice
- 1 TBSP of good-quality olive oil
- Good-quality salt and pepper to taste
- 4 x 160 g salmon fillets

Optional:
- 1 TBSP of nutritional yeast flakes

METHOD:

1. Preheat the oven to 180°C and line your baking dish with baking paper.
2. Place all the ingredients for your crust into a food processor and blend into a rough paste.
3. Place your fish fillets on your baking dish and cover with your nut and herb mixture, pressing it firmly onto the fish.
4. Bake your fish for 20 minutes or until its crust is golden and the fish is cooked. Note that baking times may vary depending on the thickness of your fish fillets.
5. Enjoy with a fresh salad, yummy-licious vegetables or both.

ENERGISING BREAKFAST PANCAKES

MAKES: 2 LARGE (4–5 SMALL) PANCAKES

INGREDIENTS:

- 1 cup of raw buckwheat, milled into buckwheat flour
- 1 tsp of gluten-free baking powder (make your own with brown rice flour, cream of tartar and bicarbonate of soda)
- 1 tsp of pure vanilla bean, ground
- 1 tsp of cinnamon
- Pinch of salt
- 2 eggs, free-range, hormone and antibiotics-free, organic eggs
- 1–2 TBSP of rice malt syrup
- 1 cup of fresh almond milk (no added sugar)
- Coconut oil to bake pancakes

METHOD:

1. Mill your raw buckwheat groats and add gluten-free baking powder, spices and salt, eggs, rice malt syrup and milk and mix altogether until well combined.
2. Leave aside for 5–10 minutes if you can (I have to confess that I personally never allow my batter this time of rest...mine almost always hits the pan straight away).
3. Heat the oil in a frying pan of your choice, pour in the batter evenly and cook over low heat for 5–8 minutes or until done on one side, flip over and cook until golden brown on other (takes another 3–5 minutes).
4. Serve with a dollop of coconut cream, fresh or frozen berries and a handful of chopped nuts of your choice.

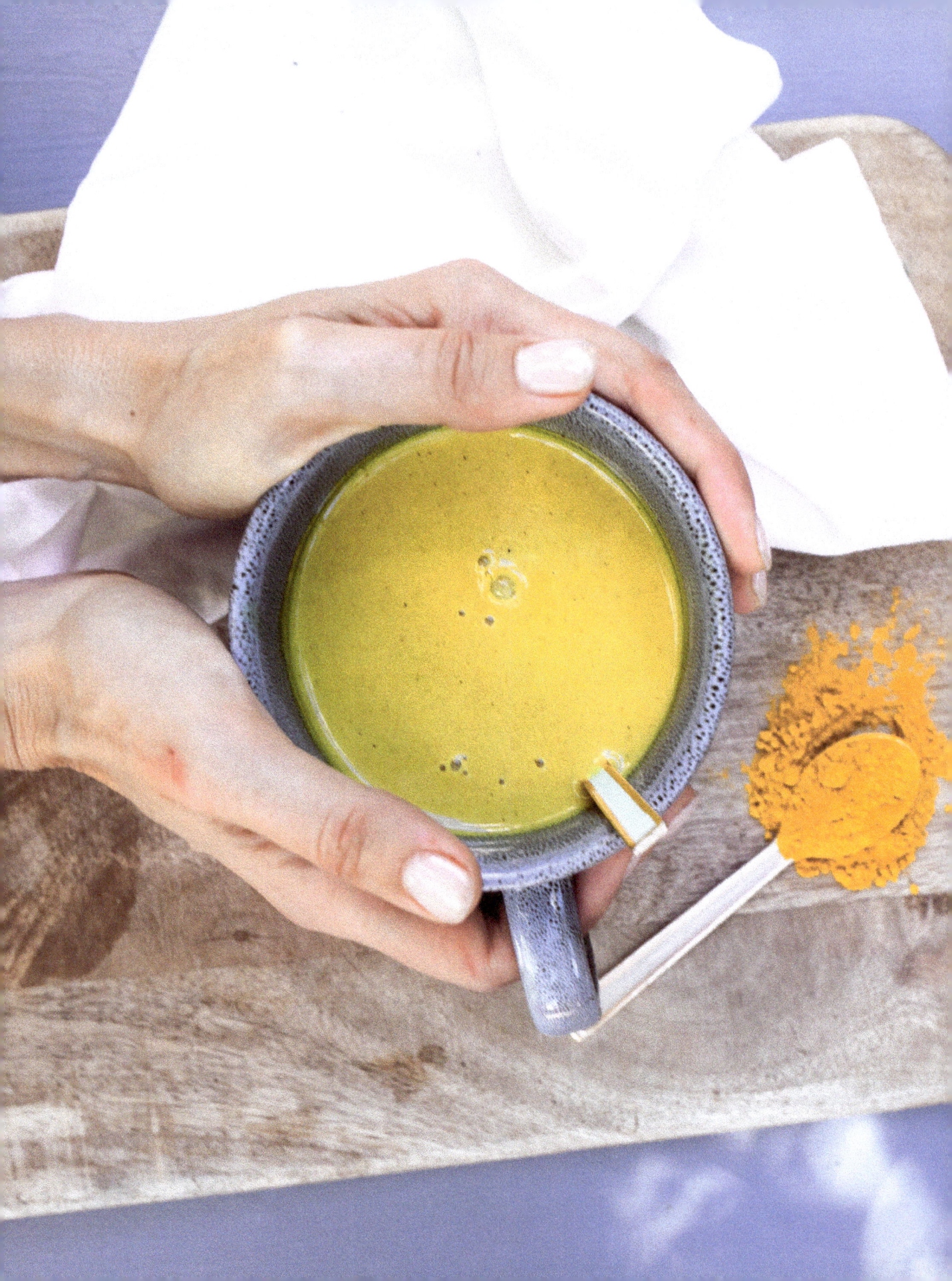

HAPPY, HEALING GOLDEN MILK

MAKES: 1 MUG

INGREDIENTS:

- 1 mug of unsweetened almond milk
- 1 tsp of turmeric powder
- ½ tsp of cinnamon, ground
- ½ tsp of pure vanilla bean, ground
- 1 small knob of fresh ginger or ¼ tsp ground
- Pinch of black pepper
- 1–2 tsp of rice malt syrup (depending on size of your mug)

METHOD:

1. Add your almond milk, rice malt syrup and spices to a small pot and bring to a simmer on low heat.
2. Be sure to whisk frequently so all your spices combine well and your milk becomes well infused with them.
3. Heat until milk is hot and has a creamy consistency.

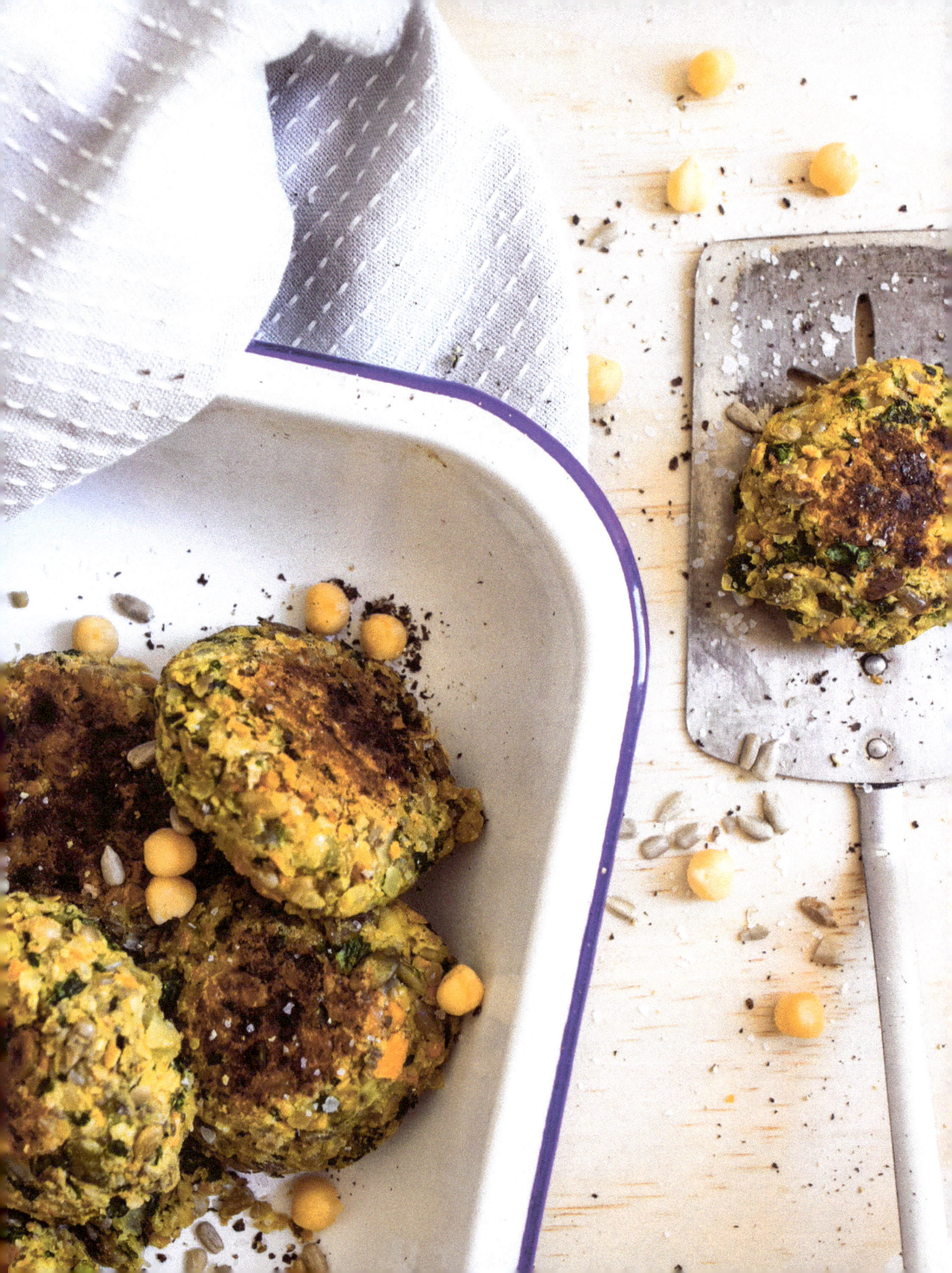

MAKE-MY-DAY CHICKPEA BURGERS

MAKES: 6 PATTIES

INGREDIENTS:

- 1 TBSP of good-quality olive oil
- 1 small brown onion, diced
- 1 clove of garlic crushed
- 1 can of chickpeas, rinsed and drained
- 1 small carrot
- 1–2 stalks of kale, de-stemmed and ripped or cut into pieces
- 1–2 stalks of celery
- ½–1 tsp of ground cumin
- ½–1 tsp of ground coriander
- 1 cup of mixed seeds (chia, sunflower, flaxseeds)
- Good-quality pepper and salt to taste
- 1–2 TBSP of good-quality olive oil for frying (alternatively bake in oven)

METHOD:

1. Put your olive oil into your frying pan and heat the onion until fragrant and soft then add the garlic and sauté for another minute.
2. In the meantime, grate your carrot and cut your kale.
3. Put your rinsed and drained chickpeas, grated carrot, cut kale, onion, garlic and mixed seeds into your food processor. Add your spices and blitz until all ingredients are well mixed.
4. Divide your mixture into little balls and flatten them a little.
5. Use 1–2 Tbsp or extra virgin olive oil to fry your chickpea patties for 5 minutes on either side or until golden brown and smelling irresistibly (alternatively bake in pre-heated oven on 180°C for 15–20 minutes or until done).

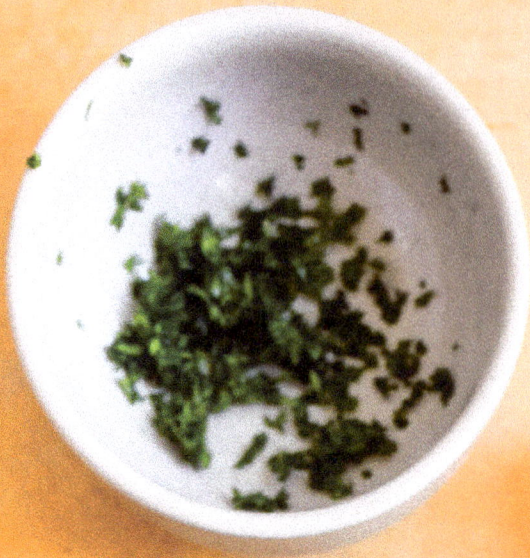

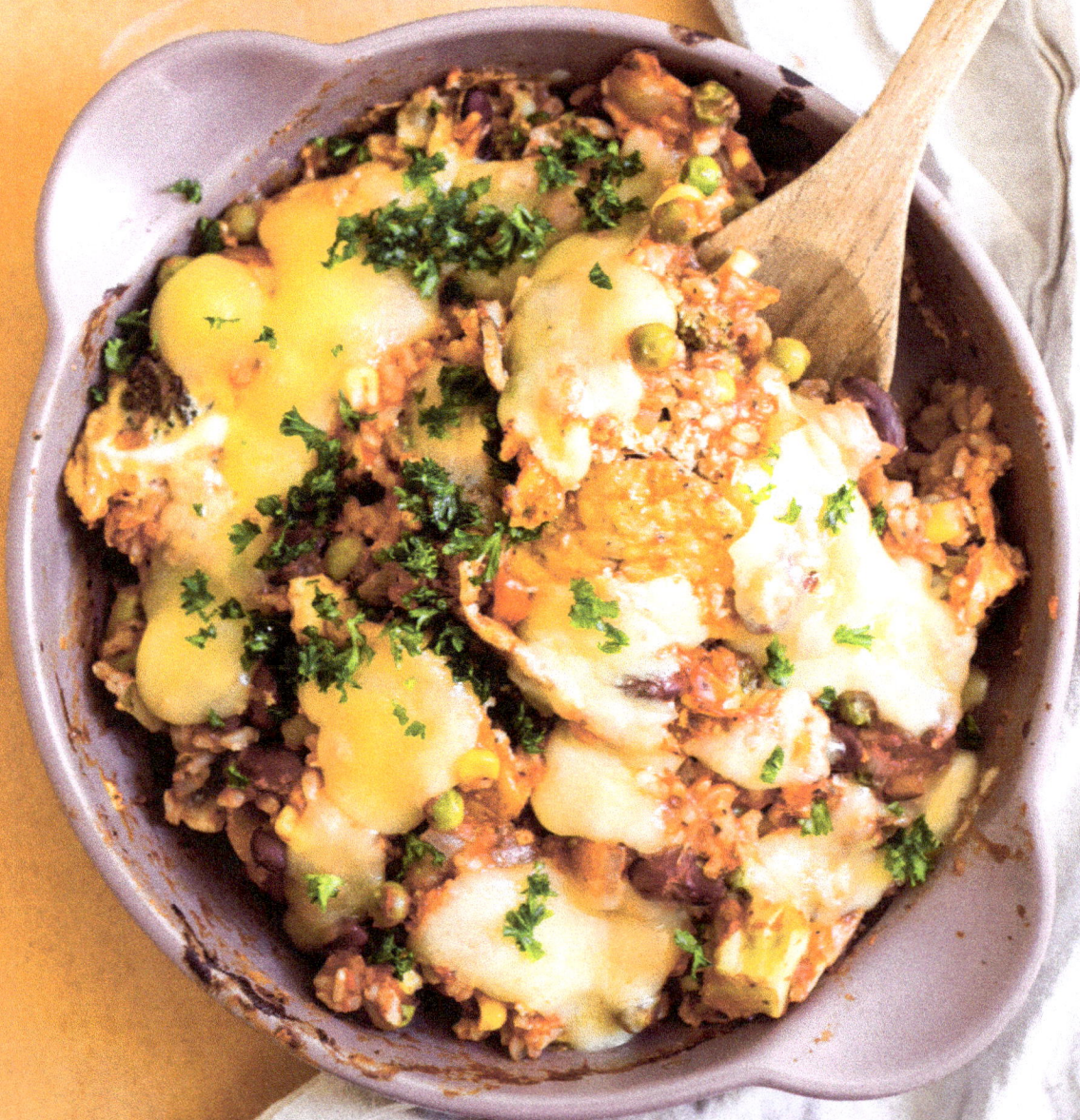

QUINOA/RICE BAKE WITH BROCCOLI AND KIDNEY BEANS

MAKES: 6 PORTIONS

INGREDIENTS:

- 1 cup of uncooked quinoa or brown rice, rinsed and drained
- 1.5 cups of good-quality vegetable stock
- 1 medium-sized onion, diced
- 2 cloves garlic, minced
- 1 cup of mushrooms, sliced
- 1 small head of broccoli, de-stemmed and cut into little florets
- ½ red capsicum, cubed
- 1 cup of garden peas, frozen
- ½ cup of corn, frozen
- 400 g or 1 tin of red kidney beans, thoroughly rinsed and drained
- 3.5 cups of tomato paste or diced tomatoes, drained
- 1–2 tsp dried oregano
- 1–2 tsp dried basil leaves
- Good-quality salt and black pepper
- 2 eggs
- ¾ cup of almond milk or yoghurt
- 1.5 cups of shredded cheese, if using
- 1 TBSP of chopped fresh parsley

METHOD:

1. Pre-heat your oven to 180°C and spray your baking dish lightly with oil.
2. Cook your quinoa/brown rice in a small pot with 1.5 cups of good-quality vegetable stock until fluffy and no water is left.
3. In the meantime, in a large pan, heat the olive oil and cook onion and garlic until fragrant. Add mushrooms, broccoli, capsicum and frozen vegetables and cook for about 3–5 minutes or until slightly underdone and still crunchy.
4. Add the cooked quinoa/brown rice, rinsed and drained beans, tomato paste or tomatoes, herbs and pepper and combine well.
5. Remove from the heat and transfer into your prepared baking dish.
6. In a cup or little bowl, mix together your eggs and almond milk. Season with good-quality salt and pepper to taste if you are not using cheese on top.
7. Sprinkle with cheese (optional) and bake for 30 minutes or until golden brown and crispy.
8. Top with fresh parsley just before serving.
9. Enjoy with a beautiful fresh salad.

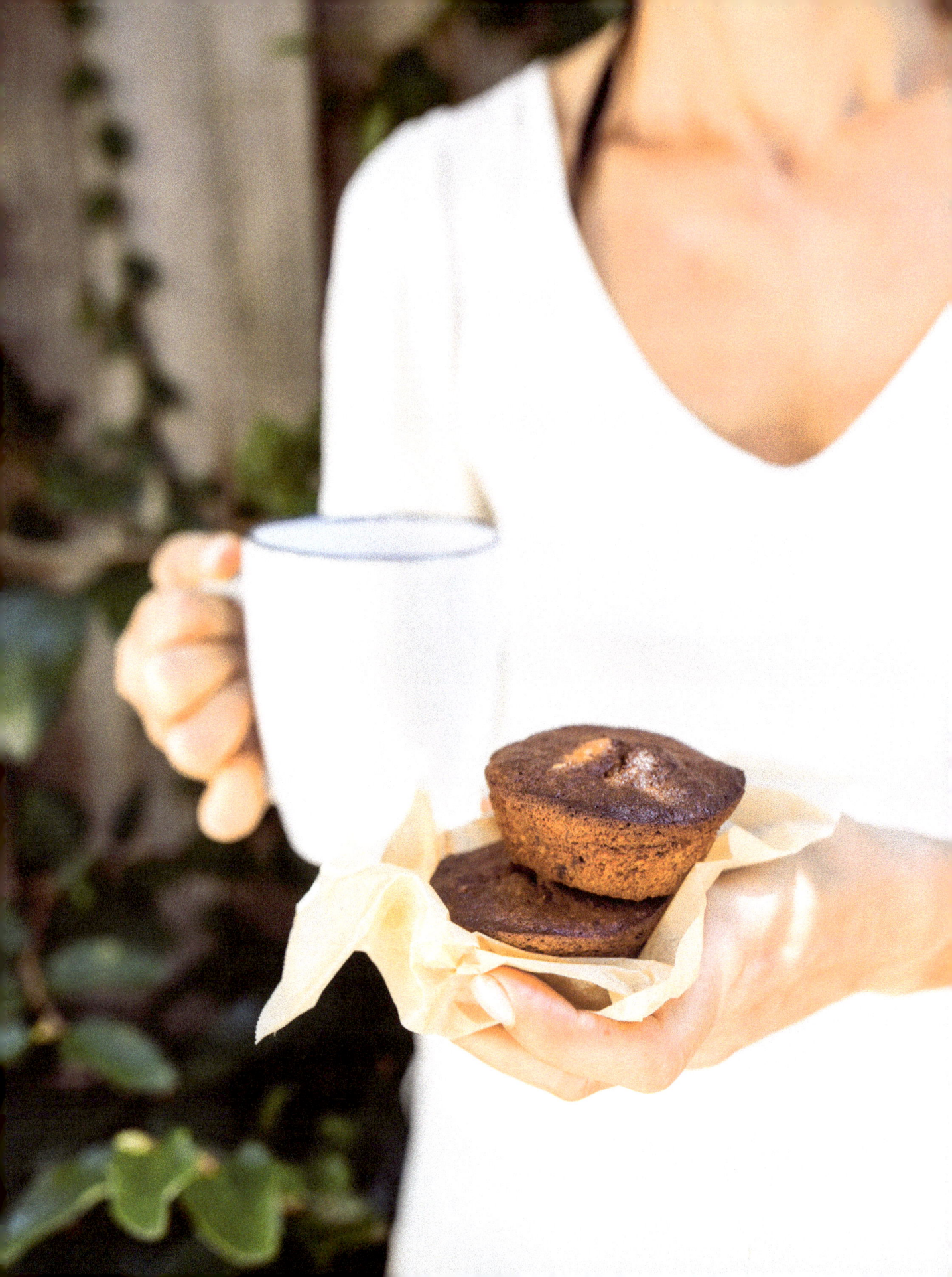

QUICK YUMMY-LICIOUS CHOCOLATE BANANA MUFFINS

MAKES: 12 LITTLE MUFFINS

INGREDIENTS:

- 1 cup of almonds, raw, blitzed into fine almond meal
- ½ cup of rolled oats
- ¼ cup of raw cacao powder, unsweetened
- ½ tsp of baking powder, gluten-free (make your own with cream of tartar and baking soda)
- ½ tsp of cinnamon, unsweetened, ground
- 1 tsp of pure vanilla bean, ground
- 1 little pinch of nutmeg, ground
- 1 little pinch of good-quality salt
- 2 ripe bananas, mashed
- ¼ cup of coconut oil, liquid
- ¼ cup of rice malt syrup
- 2 eggs, free-range, organic

METHOD:

1. Preheat oven to 180°C and grease your muffin tins with coconut oil.
2. Blitz your almonds and mix with the rest of all your dry ingredients.
3. In a separate bowl, mix all your wet ingredients together.
4. Pour your wet ingredients into your dry ingredients and combine.
5. Spoon your mixture into your prepared baking dish and bake for about 30 minutes or until done. You will know by its irresistible smell when your yummy-licious chocolate banana muffins are ready!

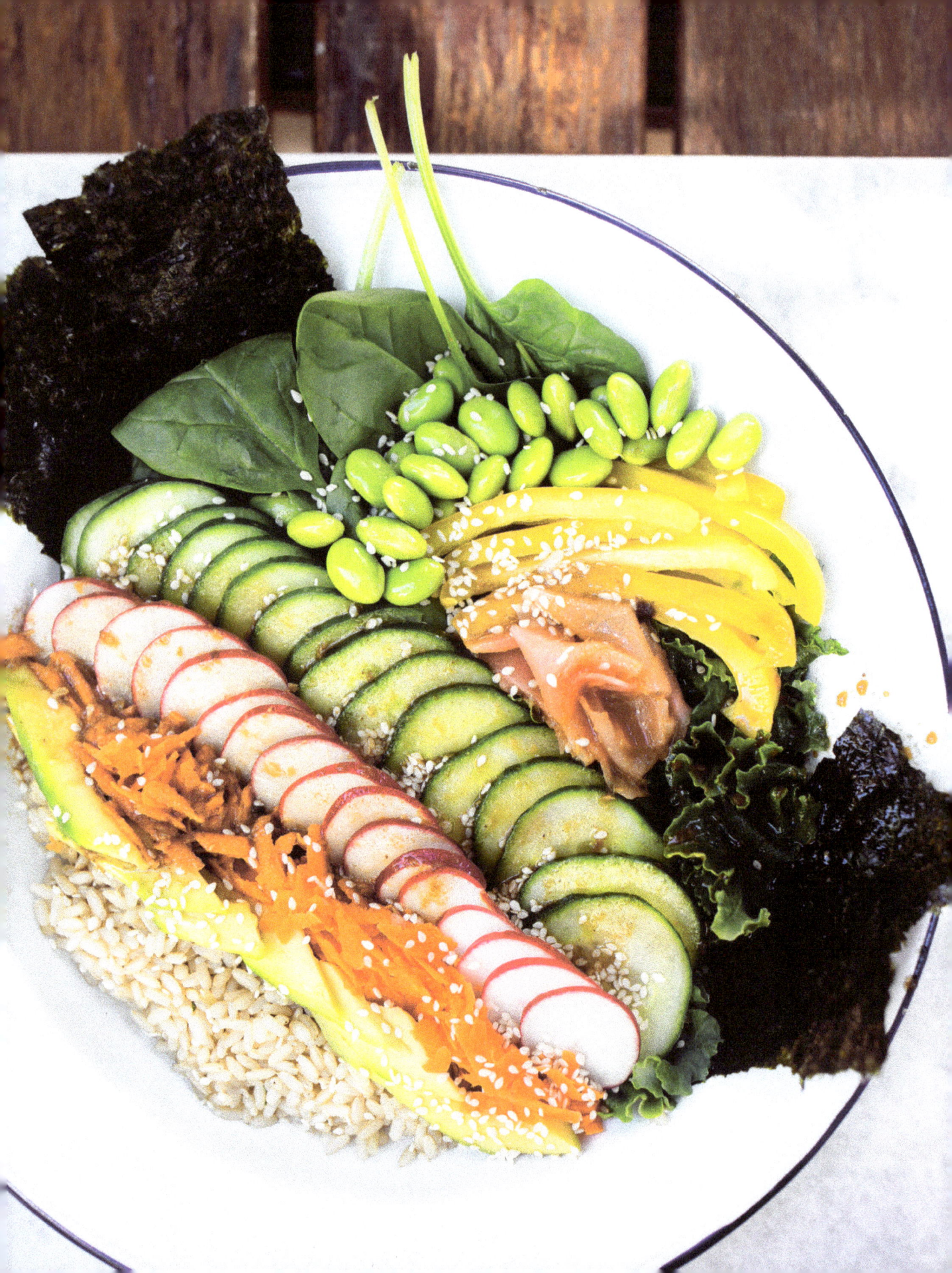

RAINBOW SUSHI SALAD BOWL

MAKES: 2 RAINBOW SUSHI SALAD BOWLS (generous serves)

INGREDIENTS:

FOR THE SALAD:

- 1 cup of short-grain brown rice, rinsed
- 1 Lebanese cucumber, washed and thinly sliced
- 1 carrot, grated
- ½ yellow capsicum, washed, seeds removed and thinly sliced
- 4 radishes, washed and thinly sliced
- 1 avocado, pitted, peeled and thinly sliced
- 4 Nori sheets, quartered and cut into thin strips
- 1 cup of shelled edamame (frozen is okay)
- ¼ cup of spring onions, thinly sliced
- 2 cups of spinach leaves
- 2 cups of kale leaves
- 2 TBSP of white sesame seeds
- 2 TBSP of black sesame seeds
- Optional:
- 1 medium slice of raw salmon fillet, cut into cubes
- or 100 g of smoked salmon, torn into bite-sized pieces

DRESSING:

- 4 TBSP of cold-pressed sesame oil or, alternatively, olive oil
- 1.5 TBSP of wasabi paste
- 4 TBSP of salt-reduced tamari sauce
- 2 TBSP of lemon juice
- 4 TBSP of apple cider vinegar
- 1 TBSP of rice malt syrup
- 1 tsp grated fresh ginger

METHOD:

1. Rinse the brown rice using a fine-meshed strainer and pour the rice into a pot. Add 2 cups of filtered water and bring to the boil. Reduce the heat and simmer until your rice is cooked and no water is left.
2. Boil your edamame beans for about 5 minutes or until bright green. Rinse and set aside.
3. Meanwhile, prepare all your raw vegetables: thinly slice your cucumber, capsicum, radishes, avocado and spring onion; grate your carrot and ginger.
4. Quarter and slice your Nori sheets and in a small bowl prepare your dressing by mixing all the ingredients together.
5. To assemble your salad, put your spinach and kale leaves at the bottom of a large bowl, then add your cooked rice and prepped vegetables. Add your Nori sheets, edamame and salmon (if using). Drizzle over your dressing and gently stir to combine. Top with sesame seeds.

IMMUNE-BOOSTING CURRY WITH SWEET POTATOES AND CHICKPEAS

MAKES: 2 PORTIONS

INGREDIENTS:

- 1 medium-sized onion, diced
- 1 TBSP coconut oil
- 2 cloves of garlic
- 1 small knob of fresh ginger, grated
- 2 tsp turmeric powder
- 1 tsp cumin seeds
- 1 tsp ground coriander
- ½–1 tsp chilli powder or flakes
- 1 can chickpeas, thoroughly rinsed and drained
- 1 large sweet potato, peeled and diced
- 3–4 TBSP tomato paste
- 3–4 TBSP coconut cream
- Good-quality salt and black pepper to taste
- 3–4 cups of kale, de-stemmed, washed and cut into large pieces
- 1 TBSP chopped fresh parsley

METHOD:

1. Heat your coconut oil in large pan or wok. Add diced onion and sauté until translucent.
2. Add your garlic cloves, ginger and other spices and heat until fragrant.
3. Add your rinsed and drained chickpeas, sweet potato cubes, tomato paste and coconut cream.
4. Cover and simmer until the sweet potato is tender (about 20 minutes). Taste and add more spices if needed. Add salt and pepper to taste.
5. Add kale and simmer for another 4–5 minutes over low heat.
6. Throw in fresh parsley just before serving.
7. Enjoy with quinoa, millet, brown or cauliflower rice.

REJUVENATING SUPERFOOD SALAD

MAKES: 2–3 PORTIONS

INGREDIENTS:

SALAD:

- 2 cups of kale, de-stemmed and thinly sliced
- 1 cup of spinach leaves
- 1 cup of rocket leaves
- 1 tin of organic black beans, thoroughly rinsed and drained
- ¼ head of red cabbage, thinly sliced
- ¼ head of green cabbage, thinly sliced
- 1 avocado, diced
- 2 oranges, peeled and diced
- 1–2 spring onions, thinly sliced
- 1 cup of parsley
- ½ cup of walnuts, raw
- ½ cup of pepita seeds
- 1 cup of herbs (I love adding mint, parsley or coriander)

DRESSING:

- 3 TBSP of freshly squeezed orange juice
- 2 TBSP of freshly squeezed lemon juice
- ¼ cup of cold-pressed flaxseed or linseed oil (alternatively use cold-pressed olive oil)
- 2 TBSP of apple cider vinegar
- 1 TBSP of Dijon mustard
- 1 garlic, crushed
- 1 TBSP of grated ginger
- Good-quality salt and black pepper to taste

METHOD:

1. Wash, de-stem and slice your kale and put in a large bowl.
2. In a small bowl, mix your dressing. Use about 1/3 of your dressing and massage into your kale until soft.
3. Pour any leftovers back into your dressing bowl and set aside.
4. Prepare the rest of your greens and add to your big salad bowl.
5. Thoroughly wash and dry your black beans, thinly slice your red and green cabbage, cube your avocado, peel and cut your oranges and thinly slice your spring onions. Add into your salad bowl.
6. Prepare your herbs and top your salad with nuts, seeds and herbs.
7. Pour your prepared dressing over your salad and enjoy!

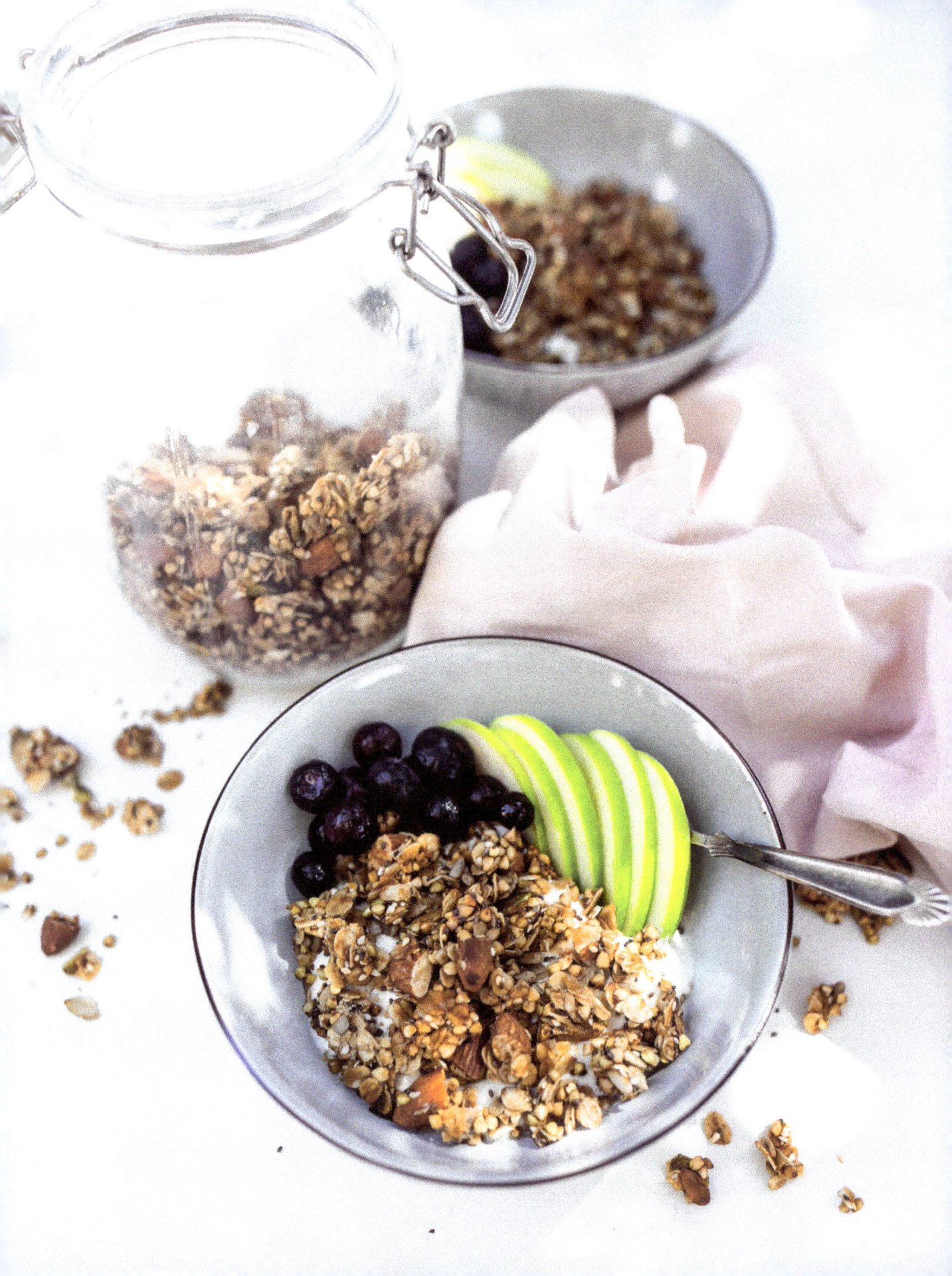

RISE AND SHINE - BREAKFAST GRANOLA

MAKES: 8

INGREDIENTS:

- 1 cup of rolled oats (for a gluten-free version: use quinoa flakes instead)
- 1 cup of raw buckwheat groats
- ½ cup of raw almonds, coarsely chopped
- ¼ cup of raw sunflower seeds
- ¼ cup of raw pepita seeds
- 1 TBSP of raw sesame seeds
- 2 TBSP of chia seeds
- ½ tsp of ground cinnamon powder, unsweetened
- 1 tsp of ground pure vanilla bean or paste, unsweetened
- Generous pinch of good-quality fine sea salt
- 3 TBSP of virgin coconut oil
- 3 TBSP of rice malt syrup
- Optional: ¼ cup of dried cranberries, unsweetened

METHOD:

1. Preheat oven to 150°C and line your baking dish with baking paper.
2. In a big bowl, mix all your dry ingredients (except your ground vanilla bean, if using) until well combined.
3. In a little pot, heat your coconut oil and rice malt syrup until liquid; add your ground vanilla bean or paste and combine well.
4. Add your wet ingredients into your bowl and mix well until every nut, seed, oat, cranberry (if using), and buckwheat groat is well coated.
5. Spread your granola mixture thinly and evenly onto your prepared lined baking tray and bake for about 30–40 minutes or until golden brown and smelling irresistible.
6. Let the granola cool completely before storing in an airtight container (keeps for 1–2 weeks stored in an airtight container in the fridge or for up to 3 months in the freezer).
7. Serve with fresh fruit such as berries and your choice of nut-milk or natural Greek-style yoghurt.

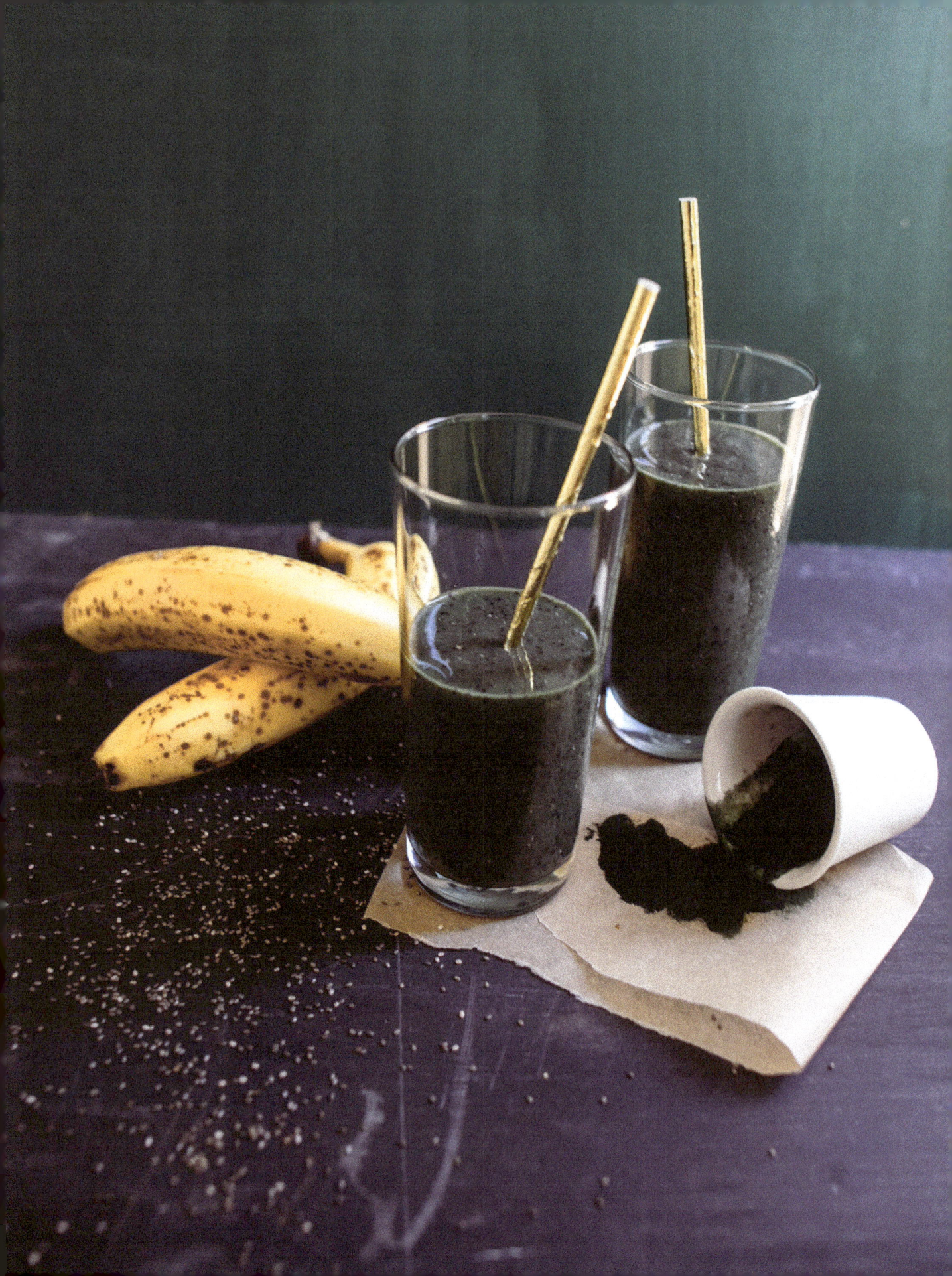

THICK TROPICAL SPIRULINA SMOOTHIE

MAKES: 2 MEDIUM-SIZED SMOOTHIE JARS

INGREDIENTS:

- ½–1 small banana, fresh or frozen
- 1 cup fresh or frozen mango pieces
- 1 cup of fresh or frozen blueberries
- 1 cup of kale, destemmed and cut or ripped into little pieces
- 1 tsp spirulina powder
- 1 TBSP chia seeds
- 1 cup of almond milk, unsweetened
- 1 cup of ice-cubes (optional, if you have been using frozen fruit, you might find your smoothie cold and thick enough without adding the additional ice cubes)

METHOD:

1. Put your fresh or frozen fruit into your high-speed blender. Add kale, spirulina powder, chia seeds, almond milk and ice-cubes, if using, and blend for 120 seconds or until you have created a rich creamy consistency and all your ingredients are well mixed.
2. Pour your health-boosting and beautifying smoothie into a pretty jar or glass and take the time to mindfully enjoy how delicious wholesome healthfulness can taste!

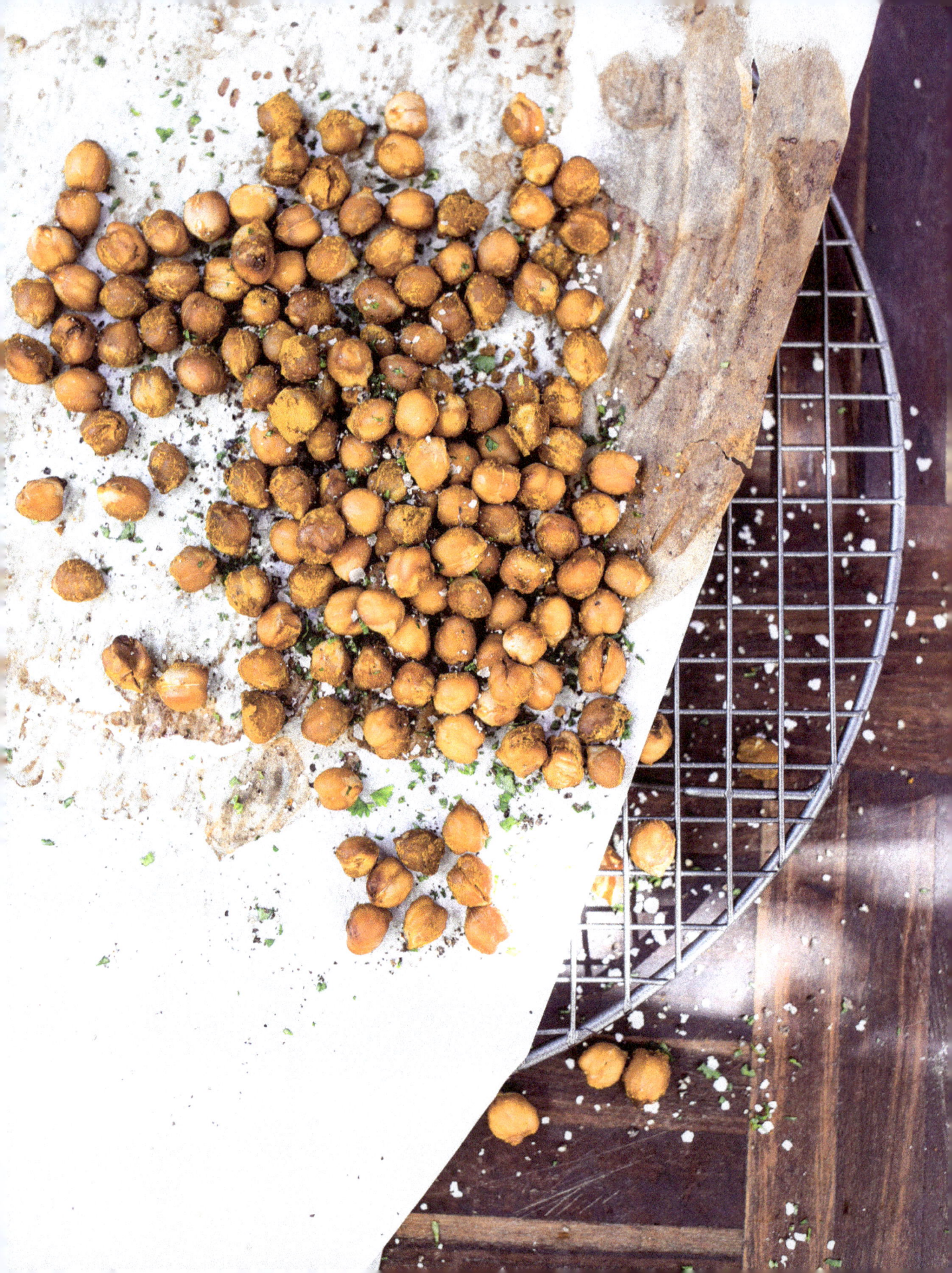

SPICY ROASTED CHICKPEAS

MAKES: 1.5 CUPS

INGREDIENTS:

- ½ cup of dried organic chickpeas (soaked overnight or for at least 8 hours and thoroughly rinsed) or 1 tin of organic chickpeas, unsalted (thoroughly rinsed and drained)
- 3 TBSP of good-quality apple cider vinegar (with mother)
- 3 TBSP of salt reduced tamari sauce
- 1 tsp of ground turmeric
- 1 tsp of ground cumin powder
- ¼ tsp of cayenne pepper
- ¼ tsp of black pepper

METHOD:

1. If using dried chickpeas soak, rinse and cook these according to cooking instructions.
2. Preheat the oven to 180°C.
3. Place all your ingredients in a little bowl and mix.
4. Coat your chickpeas well in the mixture.
5. Transfer coated chickpeas to baking try lined with baking paper.
6. Bake for 4560 minutes (depending on power of your oven) or until golden brown and crunchy.

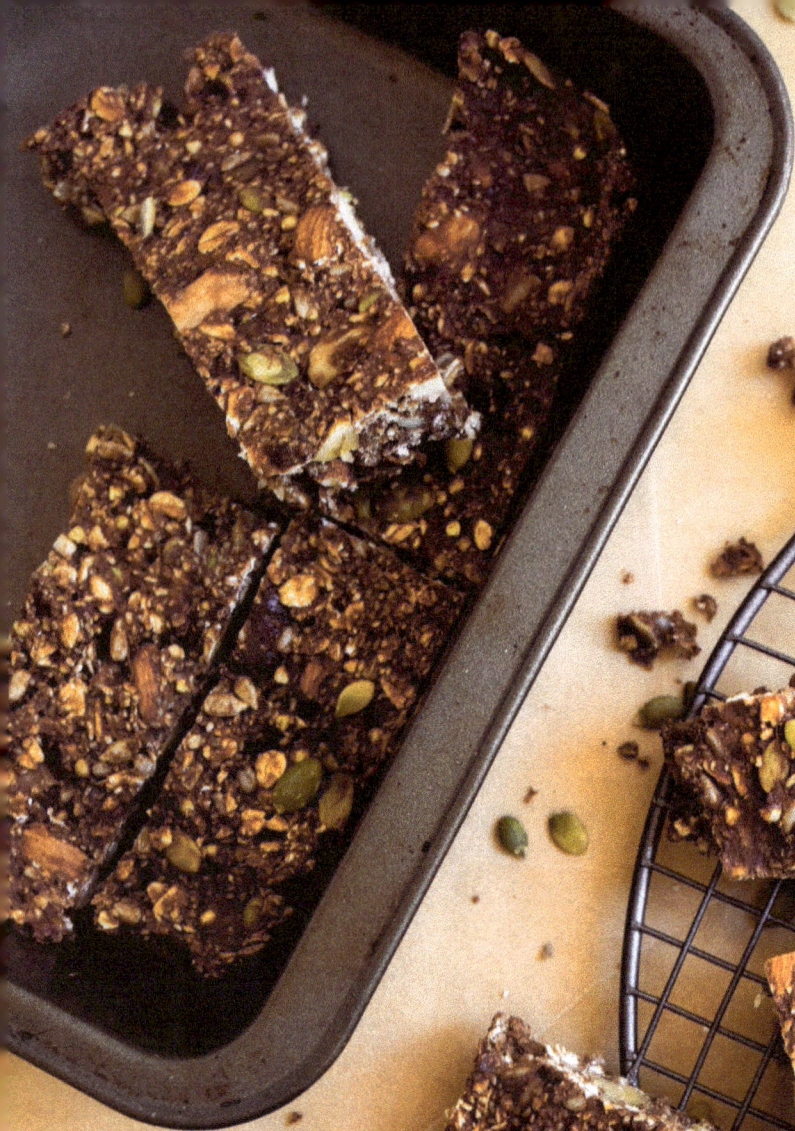

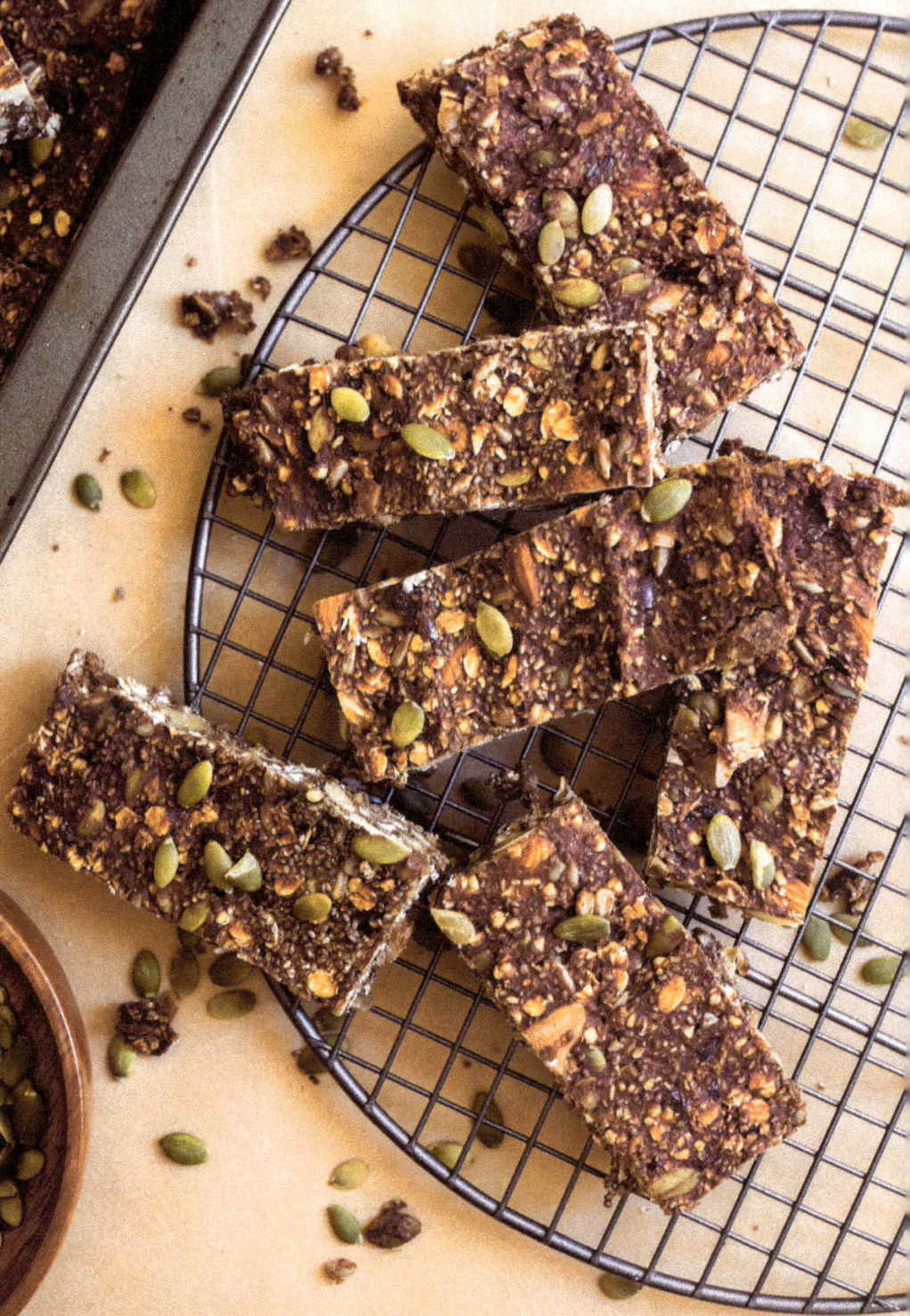

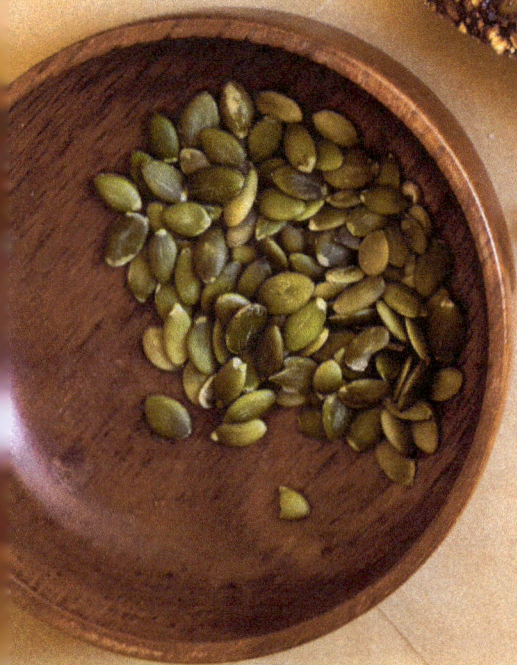

UP-YOUR-GLOW CHOCOLATE BARS

MAKES: 12 CHOCOLATE BARS

INGREDIENTS:

- ¼ cup of chia seeds – soak in just enough water to cover seeds for about 15 minutes or until all gooey
- 3 large ripe bananas, ripped or chopped into large pieces
- 1/3 cup of cacao powder, raw and unsweetened
- ¾ cup of dried Medjool dates, pitted and chopped
- 1 tsp of ground pure vanilla bean
- 1 tsp of cinnamon
- pinch of good-quality salt
- ¼ cup of tahini or almond butter
- 1 cup of rolled oats
- ½ cup of buckwheat groats
- ½ cup of shredded coconut, unsweetened
- 1 cup of mixed seeds (sunflower, pepita, sesame...)
- 1 cup of mixed nuts, raw unsalted (almonds, walnuts, hazelnuts...)

METHOD:

1. Preheat oven to 150°C (I am using low heat here and prefer to bake for longer to ensure good quality fats and amino acids in nuts and seeds are staying intact and are not being transformed) and line your tray with baking paper.
2. Soak your chia seeds in water until gooey gel forms.
3. Process your banana, cacao powder, spices, salt, cacao powder, chia seed mixture and tahini or nut-butter until smooth.
4. Mix in your rolled oats, buckwheat groats, mixed seeds, nuts and shredded coconut by hand.
5. Pour your mixture into a square baking dish and spread out evenly.
6. Bake for 50–60 minutes or until golden brown on edges and crisp. Allow to cool before cutting into little bars (keeps for up to 7 days in fridge and freezes up to 6 months).

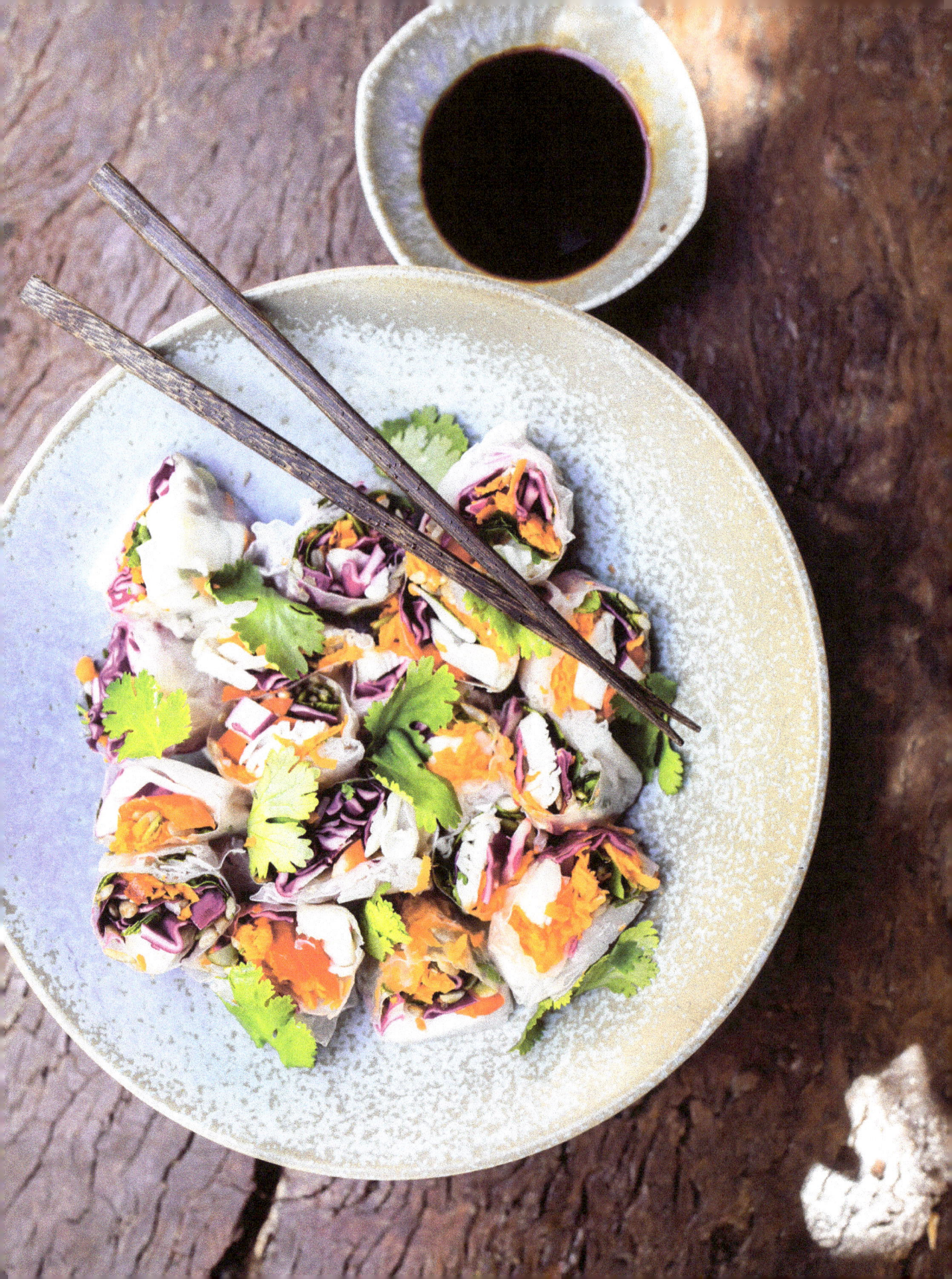

WAIST-SLIMMING RICE PAPER POCKETS

MAKES: 20 HALVES

INGREDIENTS:
- 2 large carrots, grated
- ¼ head of red cabbage
- ½ of red capsicum thinly shredded
- 1–2 spring onions, thinly sliced
- 1.5 cups of mint leaves
- 1.5 cups of coriander leaves
- 1 hot red chilli, fresh or dried and thinly cut
- 2/3 cup of sunflower seeds
- 2/3 cup of pepita seeds
- 10 sheets of rice paper

METHOD:
To prepare your filling:
1. Grate your carrot coarsely; shred your cabbage and capsicum. Cut spring onions and chilli into little pieces and gently tear mint and coriander leaves into smaller pieces (stems and roots removed).
2. To prepare your rice paper pockets:
3. Wet your rice paper with lukewarm water and then put on a clean, moist plate or board.

TO ASSEMBLE:
1. Put a small amount of each of your vegetables, spices and herbs in the centre of your rice paper.
2. Flip one side of the rice paper over the vegetables, fold in each side to form a pocket and then close. Rice paper will get sticky so it should hold nicely together. If not, add more water with your fingertips.
3. After having assembled all 10 rice paper pockets, cut each into half with a wet knife.
4. Enjoy with salt reduced tamari sauce.

REVITALISING GREEN MASH

MAKES: 4 SERVINGS

INGREDIENTS:

- 1-2 TBSP of extra virgin olive oil
- 1 tsp of cumin seeds
- ½ tsp of chilli powder
- 1 little knob of fresh ginger, grated
- 1 tsp of turmeric
- 4 cups of good-quality vegetable stock
- 1 cup of red lentils, soaked, rinsed and drained
- 1 cup of good-quality coconut milk, preferably additive- and preservative-free
- 1 medium-sized brown onion
- 1–2 leeks
- 2–3 stalks of celery
- 1 medium-sized head of broccoli
- 2 cups kale, de-stemmed and ripped into big pieces
- Optional: ½ green cabbage

METHOD:

1. Cook your onion and leek in olive oil until translucent.
2. Add your spices and sauté for another minute or two before adding your drained lentils.
3. Stir frequently and let your lentils soak up the flavour of the spices for another minute before adding your stock, vegetables and coconut milk.
4. Bring to a boil and let simmer for about 30–40 minutes or until most of stock has been soaked up into the vegetables. Either mash your cooked vegetables or enjoy them as they are.

PART 3:

GET MOVING

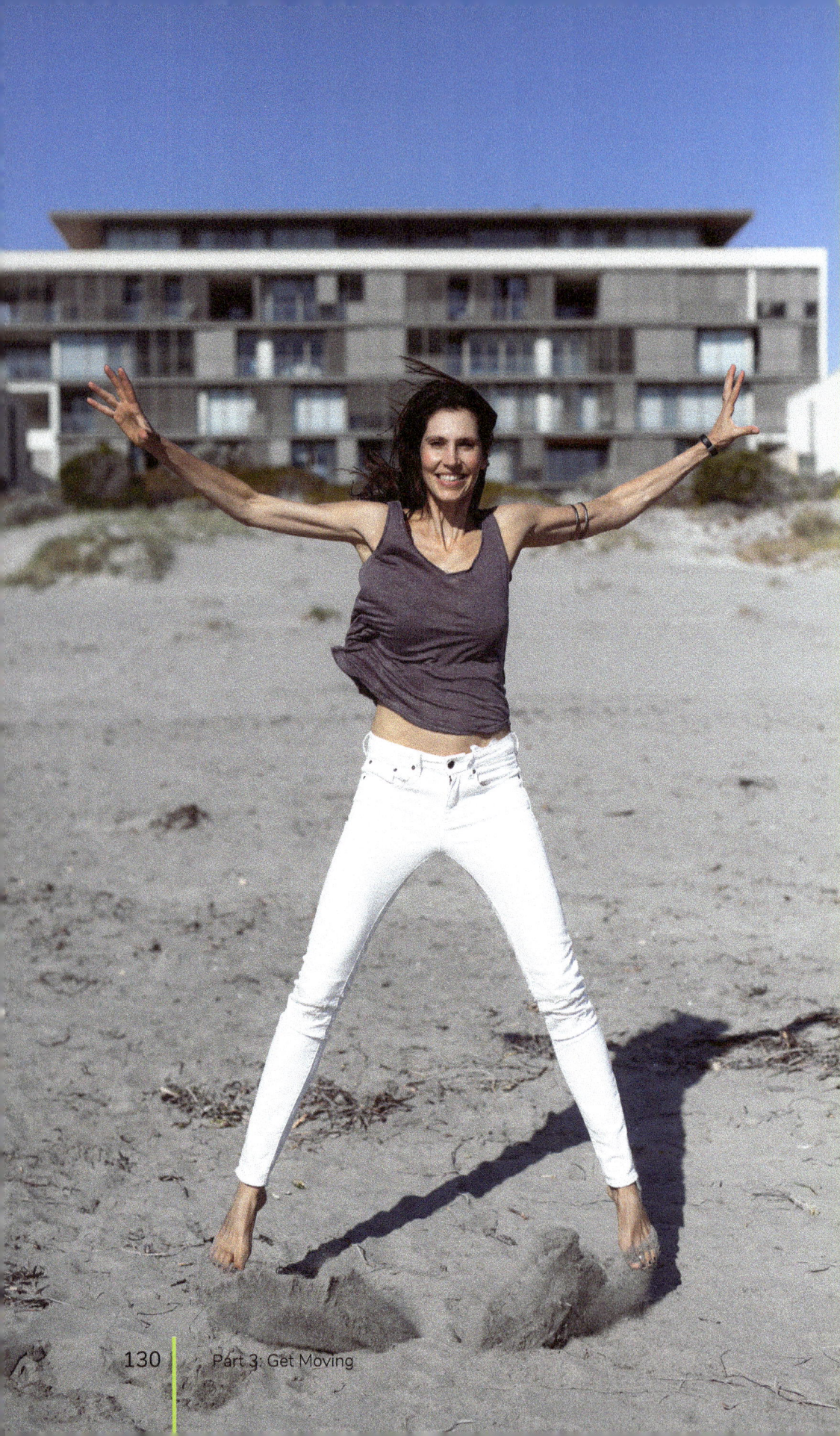

My Own Story

When I was 16, I was on summer holiday and enjoying a day with friends at the local swimming pool. Little did I know how my life was about to change. I left them at their table tennis and dived into the water. What I did not know at that time was that a vein in my brain was too thin and ready to burst any moment. The pressure exchange from the dive created that moment. I don't recall what happened in the water or how I felt, all I know is that somehow, I made it out of the pool.

On returning to my group of friends, I began feeling nauseous and really quite ill. I excused myself, telling my friends that I would meet up with them later. All at once, time seemed to shift into fast-motion. I sank to the ground and tried to crawl back to my towel. I could not see clearly and I was overcome by pain such as I had never before known. I thought my head would explode, I vomited and I remember feeling utterly powerless and helpless.

Then all of a sudden, a beam of light appeared. It approached near me and the pain drifted away. I felt lighter. A floating sense of ease and calm washed over me and all I wanted was to be one with that light.

A hard blow to my face jolted me back to reality. What the...? Had the lifeguard just slapped me?! I was outraged! I was already in such pain, such struggle, and how dare he?

My poor, bleeding brain was unable to process that he had just saved my life. The ambulance arrived and whilst being transported to the nearest hospital my ride was punctuated with impossibly loud sirens and was marked by questions too hard to answer. I remember feeling very annoyed. My name, my age, my address? Had they lost their minds? Why did they expect so much from me?

Blackness followed.

I woke up in what felt like weeks later in a hospital bed with far less brain mass and the painful realization that my body no longer performed for me the way it always had. An aneurysm stole my speech, my vision, and my ability to read and write. I could not move my body... I could not walk or talk, and I felt lost. My 16-year-old body was now governed by the brain of a very young child. The only good news was that I was still alive and that's what counted.

Whilst lying there in my hospital bed week after week, I discovered greater strength and courage than I had ever tapped into during all my years. I knew I was alive because I wanted to live. I had not given up, and I was truly fighting for my life.

On my road to recovery, it became crystal clear that it was now up to me to make the most of this amazing life and to truly grasp at my second chance. There and then, I promised myself that I would do everything I possibly could to ensure a full recovery, against all the odds, no matter what. And I did! I do not regard myself as powerful or amazing, but I made up my mind and I gave it my all, my total ALL.

As it turns out, the aneurysm was a gift to me. Having the mind of a 5-year-old again erased the teenage insecurities, angst, and false beliefs that I had adopted. The biggest gift was me giving myself permission to just go for it and make my life all it can be.

I consider myself incredibly lucky. I sometimes wonder who I might have come to be if not for this turning point. I am so grateful for my journey. I know, firsthand, how my body is both sacred and vulnerable. All that my body can do and the many magical things I had never thought to revere or appreciate can vanish in a moment. Since then, I have experienced my body's tremendous capacity for healing. And do you know what? If I can do it, anyone can do it. I am neither particularly brave nor very self-secure—I am simply an ordinary girl who went for it and my message to you is: So can YOU!!!

Whatever it is that pretends to limit you, I want you to recognise that you have the same capacity for miracles within yourself. I want you to give yourself permission to do the same. Create new fabu-licious goals for yourself. Release the self-limiting beliefs that hold you back. Take the big plunge and trust your own audacious capacity for awesomeness.

Every day our bodies do miraculous things for us, and so I invite you to view movement and motion as a beautiful celebration of what your precious body really can do. In every breath and each heartbeat, declare that your life-force is motion—it's active. I invite you to a new perspective, a new paradigm, and it is this: moving your body honours its life, its strength, and its capacity for joy, light, and love. Your body, as it is in this moment, is beautiful and perfect, as well as optimally primed to express the gift to this world that your life is.

We Are Born to Move

We are meant to move. We are built and made to propel our precious bodies forward, sideways, or up and down in one way or another. We were born to carry, lift, crawl, leap, balance, tip toe, sprint, and bend. In other words, we were born to move. This is the only way to keep our body strong and healthy through and through. It is the most powerful and efficient means to make us feel good, focused and clear. Movement clears away accumulated stress and improves all our bodily systems: from our digestive to our immune system, to our respiratory to our nervous and endocrine systems, not to mention the strength of our musculoskeletal structure. Movement beautifies us, inside and out—such as our skin, hair, nails and eyes. Are you starting to get as excited as I am about the fact that total overall health and an awesome life is all out there for you? It is available at your fingertips, simply by moving your body. I know it sounds too good to be true, but it is not. Go ahead—try it and find out for yourself.

On the opposite end of the body-moving-awesomeness-spectrum, you will find quite a different experience. Are you familiar with the dull heaviness in your body which only grows as you gradually become more sedentary? It feels like all the ease and lightness of joyful motion is suddenly being sucked out of you, replaced by tired, dull heaviness. It almost feels like we are a trapped prisoner of our own heavy body. The less we move, the more this paralysing heaviness takes control. With a dawning awareness, we realise we are aching all over. We have fallen out of tune with our own flesh and bone. We have forgotten how good we are actually meant to feel. Our bone structure is weakened and we have started to lose our graceful natural alignment—we are hunching over our desks. We slur our steps when we drag our tired bodies into elevators or cars. Are you feeling me? And the horrible thing is your mind then starts to slow down, too. Fogginess replaces mental clarity and alertness. And because you have forgotten how good movement actually feels, you think all you need is more rest. This could not be further from the truth. Just to make sure we do not misunderstand each other here—rest has its righteous place and is vitally important for being your most vibrant, gorgeous self (more on this later in part 4 of this book). But, what your body really needs right now to re-energise, rejuvenate, and rebalance is movement. To escape this exhaustion, all your body is craving is MOVEMENT. Expending energy actually attracts energy. The only way to break through this seemingly impenetrable grip of physical and mental exhaustion is by leaping into your moving action again. Walk, run, jump, ride, swim, dance, or fly—find a regular way of keeping this goddess body of yours active. It needs it because it is the only way for you to perform at your best.

And yes, I know... I hear you... All of this is easier said than done. Taking the first step to kicking off this tired heaviness feels really hard and almost un-doable. You might have convinced yourself by now that moving is simply not for you. You might also think the way you feel in your body is okay because you are not as young as you used to be. You have started tolerating this feeling of not being your best self. But this is not what I want for you. I believe this is not what you are here for. You are here on this earth to give the world the best version of yourself, to fulfil a mission only you can fulfil.

Have I always been so fit and strong and my best moving self?

The plain answer is not at all. Growing up I was long and thin with little strength and no particular sense of coordination. My mother had neither the funds to invest in developing my physical strength nor did she prioritise her own physical self. I always knew I was one of the less athletic kids and I remember dreading every kind of ball game because I felt uncoordinated and anxious about exercising in front of others. I have so much compassion for those of you who feel awkward and resistant to movement because I lived this reality, too. This is why I consider myself so very lucky and why I see the blessing in disguise. Let me be the same for you now, *your disguised, kick-ass exercise blessing*. I want you to know that anything is possible if you want it and if you commit to your gorgeous self. We can start over at any time. The only limit there is YOU (and the sky).

ARE YOU READY TO DIVE RIGHT INTO YOUR HEALTHY-LICIOUS JOURNEY?

In one quick glance, here are my top tips on how to transform yourself into a strong, radiant, glowing bombshell:

- Change begins in your mind. ALWAYS think of this journey as a privilege to nurture your precious body, allowing it to transform from dull and sluggish to a strong, agile, and radiant version of YOU.

- Start where you are. If you want to get into running but have never run before, start by integrating 5-10 small walk-runs into your walk.

- Keep a positive mindset and loving attitude toward yourself. Rome was not built in one day, either.

- Set a super clear goal and then break it down into small, do-able steps. (5-10 minutes every other day or even 3 times a week are great starting points.)

- Be realistic. When can you possibly make exercise fit into your busy life? Is it better in the morning before life gets too busy or in the evening when everything slows down?

- Allow yourself time to fall in love with it. Do it because you love how it makes you feel— empowered, awesome, healthy, thinner, stronger, as if you could achieve anything, proud of yourself, in charge, etc.

- Schedule your exercise time into your agenda as fixed appointments; block this time out.

- Create a rhythmic habit so your body will start to crave the feel-good hormones at certain times.

- Use movement YOU love and that makes YOU feel good. For example, I love nothing more than running. Even when all too often the run turns into a jog, I feel alive, free, and happy. It is during this time that my creativity kicks in. It is while I am running that I feel more focused and for that moment I feel like I can achieve anything. My body LOVES running, but your body might crave something entirely different. One of my clients loves dancing. This is when she finds the utmost pleasure and athletic worship of her amazing body. Discover what movement makes you feel alive and happy. What is it that brings out your own superwoman?

- Do not contemplate whether or not you should, but instead simply do it. Make it as routine as brushing your teeth every day. You might not be overly excited about brushing your teeth each time, but you do it anyway, knowing it is necessary for your health.

- Create accountability. Tell everyone that you have decided to change into a much fitter, stronger, and healthier version of yourself; get yourself a personal trainer or go to a group session. Having an exercise buddy can be fun and makes you accountable—knowing that someone is waiting for you has true superpowers in this regard. If you find it hard to commit to your own time, it might help to know you are also committing to someone else's time...plus it is fun to sweat together.

- Be smart when you begin. Do not overdo it as this can do two things. Firstly, it can deplete your precious energy in one go and it will set you up for failure. This transformation takes time, so break it down into manageable chunks. Only you can truly know what those bite-sized pieces of I-can-do-this will look like for you. It might mean starting with a morning meditation/breathing routine. It could also mean you are meeting your friend in the park for early morning walking with weights. It could mean you are hitting the pool after work for one lap, then two and then bit by bit adding on more lengths. And secondly, there are so many ways to start this journey of yours so do not try and do what is right for your friend or is right for me...listen to your clever self and hone into YOUR superpower and do what is right by YOU.

Do you wonder where to start? You are already in the perfect place. Begin right where you are. Your ability, your fitness level, your strength, as it is today, is absolutely perfect. Here is your GET-MOVING action-plan. Taking action will steer you right through those self-limiting beliefs.

If you lean towards a more sedentary lifestyle, begin here. If you are already a mover, skip to step two.

REDISCOVER THE INCIDENTAL MOVEMENT GODDESS WITHIN YOU

Incidental movement is simply the movement that is a natural part of your day. It is not pre-planned in a gym with a trainer, found on a YouTube channel, or streamed on a device. Try to fit as much of it as possible into your life every day.

ACTION STEPS:

1. Add a 15-minute walk into your mornings AND into your evenings.
2. Try to fit in a quick walk during your lunch break.
3. Replace the escalator or lift by taking the stairs, or even better, climb up and down them twice.
4. Dance around the kitchen.
5. Play with your kids in the park.
6. Re-paint your house.
7. Do all those repairs you have been wanting to get someone in for yourself.
8. Get up from your working desk and do 2 minutes of invigorating jumping jacks, mountain climbers, or squat jumps every time you feel tiredness creeping in on you.
9. Plank while watching TV or lengthen those beautiful tired muscles of yours with some Zen stretches.
10. Use public transportation.
11. Pull out your bike from the garage and go for a ride.
12. Intentionally, park your car on the far side of a parking lot and enjoy the walk.
13. Use technology to boost your steps. If you do not already own one, I absolutely encourage you to buy yourself a Fitbit or if you would like to go even fancier and put the money into it, invest in an Apple-watch. It is so motivating and at the same time quite shocking to see how little we move in our automated lives. No wonder our poor bodies are rebelling. Make sure you get 10,000 steps into your day. This is a recommended minimum of incidental movement per day.

My clients transform every day from fatigued, super-stressed, overworked business women and mums into happy-licious superwomen through movement. It is fair to say that with our busy, automated lives we are totally undermining the importance of everyday movement. We used to do a lot of physical labour before everything got replaced by super-efficient machinery and technology. Once upon a time, we used to walk long distances; we used to carry our baby on our backs or across the chest (or both); we used to harvest and tend to the fields. Doing every day washing used to be tough love on our muscles and making food was even labour intensive, before supermarkets and the introduction of pre-packaged food.

I am sure you would agree that life in the western world has changed dramatically over the years. What used to take a full day (laundry or making bread) can now be done in relative moments, giving us so much time freedom, so much ease, and so much comfort. I am a huge fan of modern conveniences and would absolutely hate the idea of washing all my daily loads of washing with my bare hands. Honestly!! I deeply respect the labour women performed (and still do, in some countries) every day to keep their families so well cared for. But all these marvellous technological advancements have robbed our daily experience of using our bodies for the work they were so well designed to do. Without meaningful movement, our bodies just waste away. Daily physical movement is essential to vibrant health.

So, I encourage you to take it on! Own the awesomeness you create by putting your beautiful self into motion.

What's next?

GET CLEAR WITH YOURSELF ABOUT THE JUST-FOR-YOU EXERCISE YOU CAN TRULY AND UTTERLY FALL IN LOVE WITH

"Fall in love with exercise? Is this woman crazy?" I hear you say. Yes, possibly I am crazy, but I do have a point, so hear me out. If you are looking to live your best life in your most healthy-licious body, it will be important for you to find a way of moving your body that excites you. The kind of excitement that wakes you up like you are a five-year-old on Christmas morning, so excited that it's the first thing you want to do. So excited that the initial discomfort or awkwardness is NBD (no big deal). Of course, changing from soft-bodied to fabulously fit is not easy. It is painful—newly awakened muscles trading a warm, cosy bed with a cold, out-of-breath, heart-pounding, sweaty reality aren't inclined to give up their familiar routines. It hurts!

Easing into movement takes time, and until this happens, you risk quitting before you have even really begun. This is why it is crucial to choose something that you love to do. It can take anywhere from 18 days to 254 days for people to form a new habit. Despite the common belief that change happens in just 21 days, it's possible that your body needs more time to *fall in love*.

Unfortunately, using sheer force of will to make your changes permanent is a recipe for failure. Ever wonder why your earlier efforts did not pan out, giving you the results you were after? If you are relying on your strength or willpower alone, you will reach a point where it is all too hard. When you are too exhausted to take on another day of new patterns, when you feel truly too busy and when something interrupts your new routine, if you don't love the movement that will change your life, you will simply fail again. You will prove once more that being active just is not your thing and will never be your thing. You might as well give up now, huh? Friend, let me tell you: I know this isn't true about you.

If you want a breakthrough to discovering yourself and your sexy, awesome, moving body, the only way to it is LOVE. Love yourself enough to find something that you LOVE to do. Let's set you up with wonderful feel-good-movement-success by finding the physical activity that leaves you feeling so insanely amazing that you want to get back to it. Let's find YOUR form of feel-good exercise that will unleash your total magic. Can you remember a time in your life when movement brought out the best in you? When you felt like you could achieve and do anything—like you were a new version of your former self—powerful, happy, energized, full of life and excitement. When every cell of your body was awake, vibrant with sheer joy?

How did you move that made you feel radiant and complete as a child? I invite you, at this moment, to fill your entire mind with the energy and strength you had back then. Which activities could you not get enough of and that brought the best out in you? Go back to doing exactly that. In my case, it is running. There is nothing in the whole wide world that I enjoy more than putting those sneakers on and pounding my feet onto the ground in a rhythmic flow. During the first few steps my brain is still full and weary, I am still self-conscious and totally overthinking everything, my breathing is still out of tune and my body might feel sore or heavy. However, after those first few initial steps, true magic happens—it's like my legs get wings, my body feels strong and capable, and my mind stops buzzing. I enter a world of total running bliss.

I know we are all different and it truly is important to honour who YOU are and what makes you YOU. So, while running might totally not be your thing, it's so important that you really trust your own body and find YOUR movement which brings the best out in YOU. Trust and follow your heart and find your moving bliss. And once you have found it, don't let it ever slip away from you again.

EMPOWER YOURSELF WITH KNOWLEDGE TO UNDERSTAND HOW EACH FORM OF EXERCISE NURTURES YOUR BODY

▶ Cardio versus weights versus flexibility

Exercise is not a competition. Each type of movement has a righteous place in your fit life. A healthy body needs and deserves to be strengthened by all three forms of movement to totally sparkle and be at its best. It is incredibly empowering to know how each form of movement can bless your gorgeous physical self.

Why cardio?

Cardiovascular or aerobic forms of exercise have fallen a bit from the limelight it once enjoyed. The fitness world is now almost hyper-focused on strength training. Of course, strength training is vital, but it can do only what it is designed to do. Strength training cannot deliver what cardio can, and vice-versa. The important thing about cardio work in expanding your health is that it allows your body to increase its oxygen uptake. This strengthens your heart, enabling it to more efficiently pump blood through your body. As your heart becomes stronger, you will feel more fit and less out of breath.

Cardiovascular exercise is proven to:

- Lower your bad cholesterol (the artery-clogging goo).
- Balance your blood sugar.
- Help maintain healthy blood pressure.
- Boost your self-confidence.

- Elevate your mood.
- Increase your immunity.
- Increase your mental focus.
- Strengthen your memory.
- Give you a deeper, more peaceful sleep.
- Clear and brighten your skin.
- Decrease your stress levels.
- Help with arthritis and maintain healthy joint function/range of motion.

Wow. Total magic, right?!

The examples of aerobic forms of movement are endless; you are limited only by the reach of your imagination. Here is a little creative push in the right direction for you to get out and go:

- Walking
- Running
- Hopping
- Skipping
- Jumping
- Cycling
- Soccer
- Basketball
- Netball
- Tennis
- Mountain climbing
- Bushwalking
- Skating: roller skate, roller blade, or ice skate
- Dancing
- Aerobics
- Water aerobics
- Marching with high knees

Why engage in weight-bearing exercise?
Here are some health benefits of weight lifting and strength training:

- Strengthens and tones your muscles.
- Reduces the risk of osteoporosis.
- Converts your muscle:fat ratio—more muscle, less fat
- Can prevent or improve chronic conditions, including diabetes, obesity, back pain, arthritis, and depression.
- Improves posture.
- Elevates your overall sense of well-being.
- Boosts your self-confidence.

- Makes you stronger, allowing you far better management of daily tasks, such as lifting, carrying, bending, and twisting (all things you do every day when you're parenting, managing a household, shopping, etc).
- Slows age-related cognitive decline.
- Transforms your sleep quality.
- Improves your sense of balance and coordination, preventing falls and injury.
- Increases your range of motion.
- Improves your overall stamina.

I am a big fan of body-weighted exercises for a couple of reasons: you can literally do them anywhere at any time and they are especially effective. It is so much easier to cheat with weights or on machines, but almost impossible to evade your own body weight. In saying this, real magic happens when you mix it all up and add other forms of resistance into your regime. It really is awesome, because there is no end to all the different versions of muscle strengthening exercises you can come up with. Get creative, my gorgeous friends. This is sooooo fun!

Examples of resistance training exercises:

Body-weight resistance:
- Squats
- Lunges
- Dips
- Chin-ups
- Push-ups
- Planks
    - Side-planks
    - Reverse planks
- Step ups/step downs
- Calf raises

Using free weights, kettlebells, medicine balls, and resistance bands:
- Bicep curls
- Triceps, overhead extensions or kickbacks
- External or internal shoulder rotations
- Shoulder raises
- Bent over rows
- Deadlifts
- Kettlebell swings

Using machines:
- Leg curls
- Leg press
- Leg extensions
- Leg abduction/adductions

- Chest fly
- Chess press
- Biceps curls
- External or internal shoulder rotations
- Cable rows
- Triceps press downs
- Cable cross-overs

Why work on stretching and flexibility?
- Prevents injury.
- Improves your circulation.
- Increases your mobility and range of motion.
- Improves posture.
- Reduces pain, particularly back and neck pain.
- Relieves stress.
- Boosts your athletic performance.
- Heightens your body-mind connection.
- Elevates your general well-being.
- Lengthens your muscles, preventing them from bulking up.

Great examples for stretching and improving your flexibility:
- ▶ Dynamic stretches
    - Leg swings
    - Lunges
    - Twists
- ▶ Static stretches (holding the stretch of a given muscle group)
    - Hamstrings
    - Quadriceps
    - Biceps
    - Triceps
    - Calves
    - Shoulders
    - Frontal plane stretches
        - o Side-bends
    - Sagittal plane stretches
        - o Flexion and extension moves, e.g., flexing the back in a backbend or forward fold helps keep the spine supple
    - Transverse plane stretches
        - o Rotations and twists, e.g., supine spinal twist (one of the best stretches ever to release tension around the back and glutes muscles)

Examples of some of my favourite lengthening, feel-good stretches:

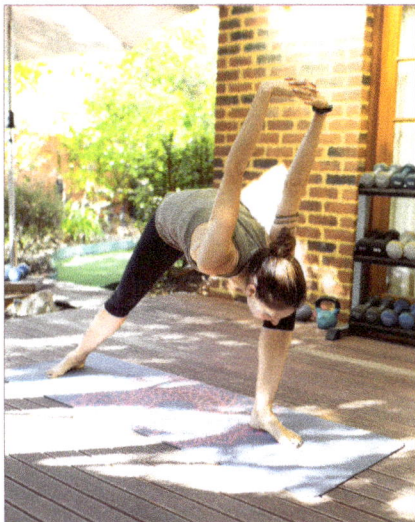

Humble warrior - stretches shoulders, arms, legs and back

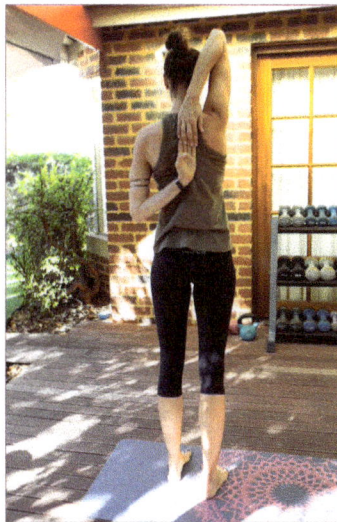

Triceps and shoulder stretch

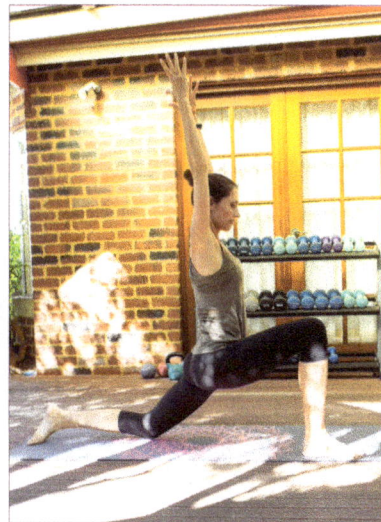

Low lunge - stretches thighs, hips, feet

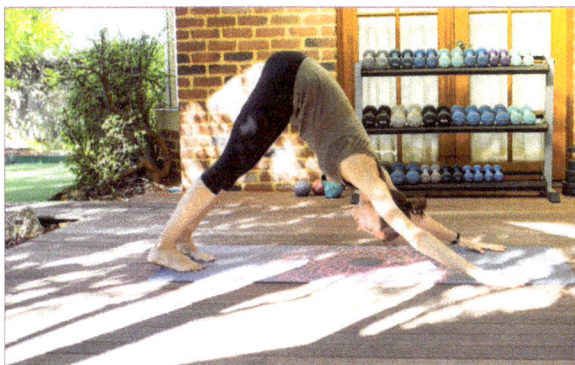

Downdog - stretches spine, hamstrings, calves

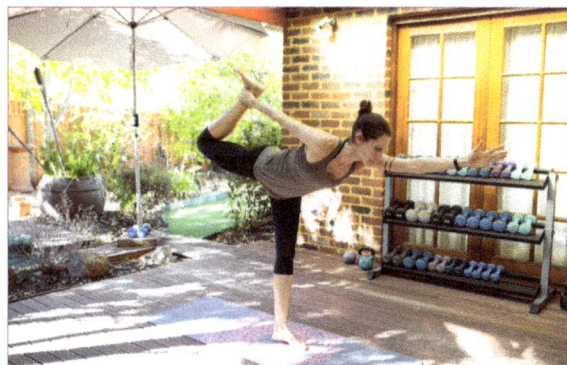

Dancers pose - balancing pose - stretches ankles, legs, thighs, abdomen, thorax, chest, hips

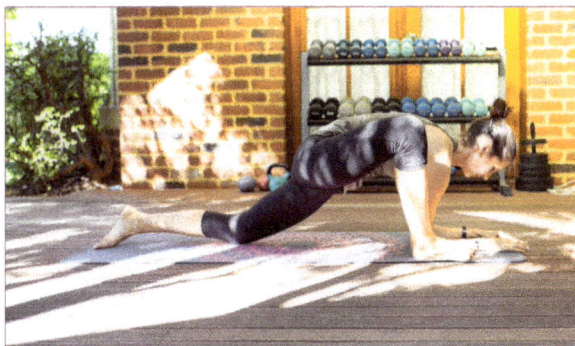

Hip flexor stretch

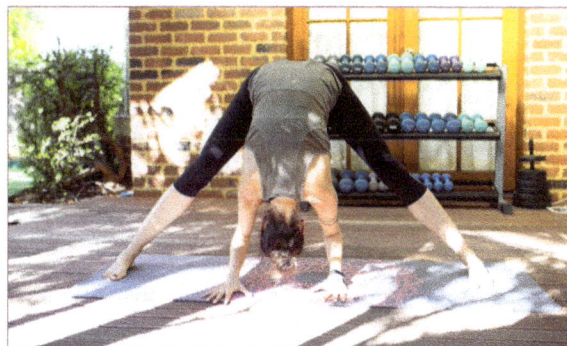

Wide forward fold - stretches hamstrings, hips, lower back, spine

In one glance: Why regular movement is your total super-power

REGULAR MOVEMENT

- **Reduces the risk of chronic diseases such as cardiovascular disease, diabetes, stroke, cancer, osteoporosis, hormonal issues, asthma, and chronic fatigue.**
- **Keeps unhealthy weight-gain in check.**
- **Makes you happy.**
- **Is like a mini-spa treatment for your skin.**
- **Gives your brain a little turbo-boost.**
- **Is like a warm hug to your self-esteem.**
- **Is your best natural energizer.**
- **Promotes deep, healing sleep.**
- **Is your most effective stress buster.**
- **Keeps your body flexible, strong and fit.**

Are you back in? Do I still have your commitment of uncovering the best, healthiest, happiest and most gorgeous version of YOU by moving daily? Great, Let's do this!

▸ **What is the right ratio of cardio to strength to flexibility for YOU?**

Do you wonder how to make this work? How many exercises and of what kind are right for you? Great question. The best answer is: "This is individual to you." It's for YOU to decide what your body needs to become its very best.

In formulating your personal ideal, consider these questions:

- ❓ What is your current physical condition?
- ❓ What is your lifestyle?
    - o In what ways are you already physically active?
    - o Does your work require aerobic activity (lots of walking)? Physical strength (lifting)? Flexibility (twisting, extending)?
    - o Is your job sedentary?
    - o Do you have small children?
    - o Do you keep animals—pets, farm/ranch animals, etc.?
- ❓ What are your goals?
    - o Do you want to strengthen and tone?
    - o Slim down and get lean?
    - o Loosen stiff muscles?
    - o Prevent back pain?
    - o Soothe knee issues?
    - o Gain flexibility?
- ❓ What do you most enjoy?
    - o Do you prefer to be indoors or outside?

o Are you social or introverted?

  o Do you prefer instruction (i.e., a personal trainer or a workout video)?

  o Do you like to be in the moment and thrive on your intuition?

❷ What are your circumstances?

  o Do you have access to a gym, a park, an outdoor track, a pool?

  o Do you have the support you need/desire?

  o Can you generate what may appear to be missing so you can succeed?

❷ What are your weaknesses?

  o If you have a heavy frame, you may prefer to lift weights rather than strain your cardiovascular system. Or, increasing your endurance may just be precisely what your body craves in order to feel happy.

❷ How can you best coordinate movement that complements the regular requirements of your everyday life?

  o A nurse who is on her feet all day might benefit more by balancing her cardio-supportive career with strength and flexibility exercises.

  o Someone who works a physically demanding job may require less strength training, but would benefit by improving their flexibility and including some moderate cardio work.

  o A person with an office job may feel drawn to balance all three areas into her healthy-licious moving life.

I encourage you to really, really listen to your body. It truly knows how much YOU will need of what, and if you listen carefully, it will tell you.

For example, if you're a regular runner, but you are experiencing shoulder pain and feel more stressed following your run, your body is gently inviting you to choose movement that better aligns with your commitment to stress-relief and pain management. It will always lead you right if you trust it and listen. Don't worry! A message to stop running now is not a message to stop running forever!

Perhaps you love heavy lifting and have made it your primary form of exercise. But lately, you have noticed that you feel more bulky than lean, which was not your goal. Your body knows this result does not balance with your desires; it is gently but intentionally inviting you to include more cardio and stretching to your movement practise. Our bodies thrive best when they are nurtured with exercises and movements that create harmonious balance in our physical lives. That is, they aim to strengthen what is weak, lift what is heavy, and bring flexibility to what is rigid.

HOW TO MAKE PHYSICAL ACTIVITY FIT INTO YOUR BUSY LIFE

1. *Prioritise.*

  ▶ I know this is not easy. In the end, we each have only 24 hours in a day. Every day demands its non-negotiables: the hours reserved for work, for parenting (lessons, school, homework, chauffeuring), and for home-making (cooking, cleaning, shopping) and then for sleeping. However, if you think about it and go over your day in your head, you will notice pockets of time interspersed throughout your day. It may be 20 minutes during your lunch break after you have eaten or an evening hour or two after the kids have gone to bed. It may be a bonus morning hour just before your kids are awake, where your husband is home and available to keep a loving watch over them while you nurture yourself.

▸ Our habits often argue against reason. Some typical objections are: You love hanging out with your colleagues at lunchtime; you look forward every day to unwinding in the evenings in front of the TV; waking up an hour earlier when you are already so tired? Who does that?

▸ If those arguments against exercise are familiar, then this is not a matter of time but a matter of priorities. And that is fine, but if you want to see and feel some change in your life and your gorgeous body, maybe it is time to shift your priorities. You know it is true. If you truly want something badly enough, you will make time for it. You will find a way, even with your crazy busy schedule. You will try getting up earlier to fit your workout into your day before your day gets the better of you. You will replace your chit chat with your colleagues with a walk or quick weights session and you will fit your yoga practise into your chilled evening.

Are there now even more little time-windows appearing in front of your inner eye where you could make movement part of your happy routine? Awesome. Keep at it. Once you start, you will come up with far more than you thought possible.

2. **Manage your time**

▸ In order to make the best use of my 24 hours, I rely very heavily on planning my day in advance. I know this might be less sexy than being super spontaneous, but it works. It gives me extra time. I put my exercise clothes out the day before and have my overnight oats in the fridge, ready to eat once I hop out of the shower. I know precisely when I am meeting clients and where my creative spaces are for creating more programs, working on a new recipe or blog, and marketing online through Facebook and Instagram. I will make these things happen without any procrastination. There is no doubt that planning ahead and being prepped keeps me sane. It's one of the reasons why I am so successful at what I am doing. It simply makes my life go around and *in flow*.

▸ I love using "The 4 Quadrants of Time Management" created by Stephen Covey. This is an absolutely brilliant strategy for prioritizing my 1001 tasks. Obviously, I prefer certain chores over others, but they do not all have the same importance or urgency. By sorting them by their importance and their urgency as he suggests, I am making sure I am not wasting my time on things that do not really allow me to move forward in the direction of my goals, such as getting sucked into a "scroll-hole" on Instagram or Pinterest.

▸ When I plan my week or day ahead, I do so by dividing all of my various duties into 4 different to-do sections. I fill my first quadrant with all the jobs that are important AND urgent, that is anything that cannot wait, but needs to be dealt with straight away (e.g., make sure I am meeting all my deadlines for all my sessions, follow-ups, reply to urgent client emails and handle all requests due that day).

▸ I reserve the next quadrant for everything that is important but not urgent. In this section I pack everything that brings me closer to my goals but does not have to show immediate (as in today) results. This quadrant provides for my long-term or intermediate-term goals and here is room for my exercise, healthy eating, and for professional development—to advance my career, improve my skills, and strengthen my mindset.

▸ Quadrant 3 provides for what is urgent but not so important, e.g., phone calls with the extended family, grocery shopping for the evening, and text messages from friends (unless they ask for immediate, life-saving support—in which case, this is moved up to Quadrant 1). I find Quadrant 3 the trickiest to get right. (I am definitely a work in progress here.) To fill this section correctly, we must learn to say "no" to others, which is often incredibly difficult for us as women. It helps me to remind myself of the fact that if I spend hours doing minor favours that make little difference in the world, I have no time to do the big stuff—that which I am here on this planet to do. My purpose and mission is to make our place happier and healthier for all of us. It is a powerful thought that gives me courage to use that little "n" word... "NO!"

▶ Quadrant 4 is for the unimportant and not so urgent. These tasks are often distractions we create to help us avoid taking action on our true purpose. Whether it's mindlessly surfing the internet, getting buried in YouTube channels, binge-watching Netflix, or deciding that today is perfect for organizing a closet you never open, Quadrant 4 really has no true demands.

▶ I hope this will empower you (as much as it empowers me) to prioritise and sort through your task list. (Thanks, Stephen, for creating such a wonderful tool to help us discover how time rich our days actually are!)

▶ Finally, don't be shy to delegate. Consider what chores and tasks on your list could be handled by someone else. What can your children do? Your partner? Perhaps giving up control of your kitchen or dinner menu might lighten your super-achiever-multi-tasking-wonder-woman workload. Just because you *prefer* your way of doing things doesn't mean you are the only one who can get that job done. Consider hiring a cleaner to handle your housework or a gardener for your yard. You could investigate the wonderful world of online shopping to save yourself a job and some time. Such decisions are deeply individual and stand really as opportunities to invest in and nurture yourself. Find your personal rhythm for designing a life that brings you your healthy-licious joy and satisfaction.

3. Win time by taking that time

▶ Let me share some true magic with you: if you take the bold step and simply exercise a few minutes at a time, you will get back minutes double-fold in your day. How is this possible? Aren't those ten, fifteen, or twenty minutes irretrievably lost? While it's true that those specific minutes are spent, it's also true that you have gained back more energy, clarity, and focus. That exercise has caused your brain to release neurotransmitters, those beloved happy hormones which, paired with energetic clarity, turns YOU into a total productivity superpower! No lie.

▶ Regard those active minutes as an investment in your gorgeous self, to set your heart right and to release those happy hormones and clear your head space. You will be a more efficient you. Trust me, you will be surprised by all the things you can get done in a very short amount of time when you have got your exercise glow on. It is not only the best time swap ever, but its most pleasant side effect creates a healthier you. Win-win! I love it, and so will YOU!!!

Are you ready to simply take this first all-empowering first step towards the new HEALTHY-licious YOU? Do it Now. Not tomorrow or the next day, and stop listening to all your insecurities which might try to convince you that it is all too hard. It is not. Deep inside you, you know it. Fact is, my beautiful warrior girlfriend, you have already dealt with far harder things in your life. The key is to take this very-scary-but-insanely-wonderful journey of transformation in little steps. One at a time. Let me take you by your hand and walk with you. Together everything is easier, don't you agree?

We are off, Beautiful!!! This is really happening!!! You are happening!!!

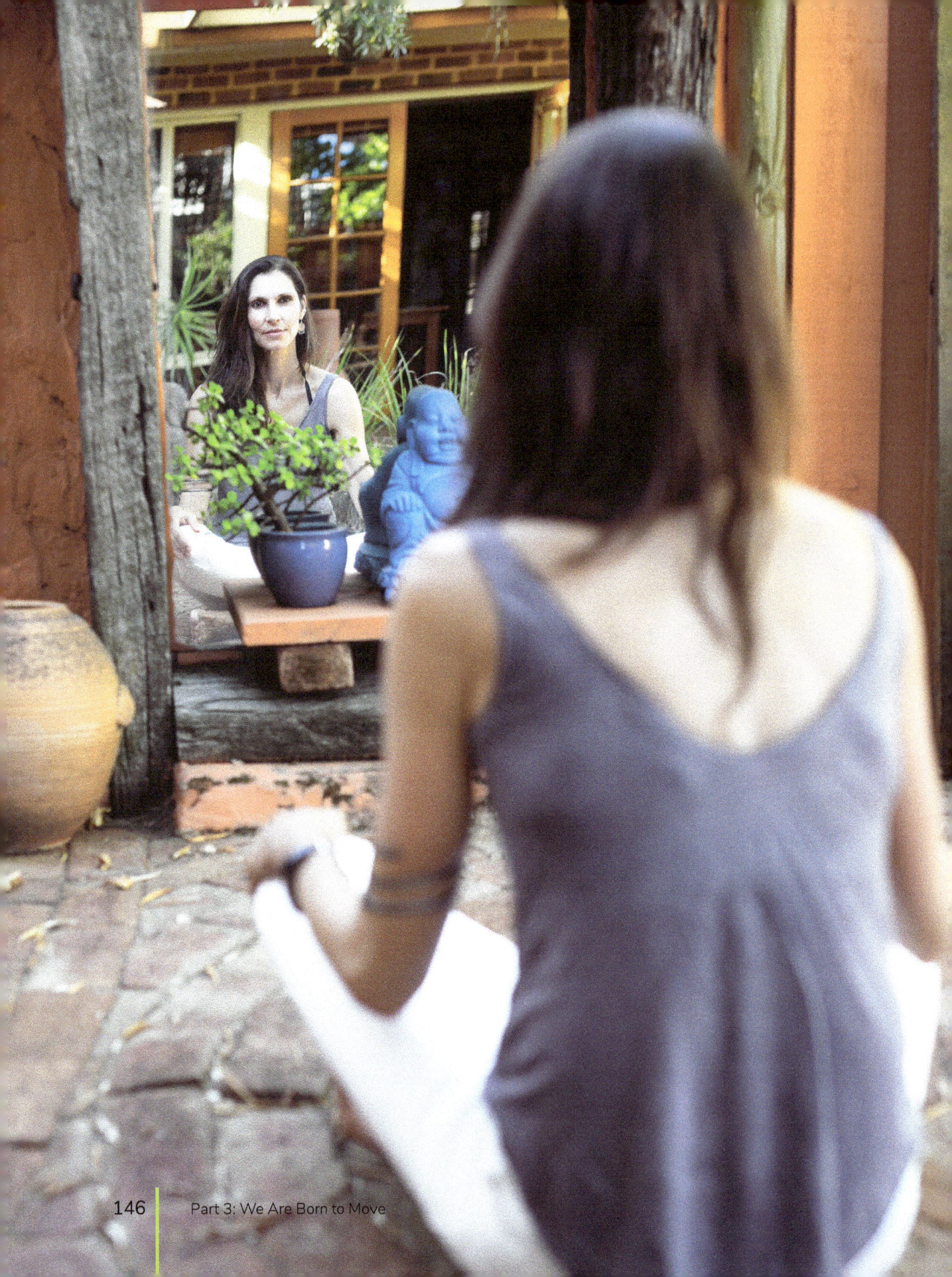

Part 3: We Are Born to Move

How to Keep Your Healthy Up

Even though this is a pretty awesome action plan to get you up and moving towards your vibrant-feel-good self, I also know that life will happen and get in your way. So, let's consider everything that could keep you away from owning this best new version of you. The clearer you are about the obstacles that might block your journey, the more capable you will be to gracefully surmount them.

OBSTACLE NUMBER 1: YOUR MOTIVATION IS RUNNING THIN

Your "honeymoon movement phase" wears off, you simply do not feel like moving, you cannot see any results yet and old patterns seem to get the better of you. Consider the following action steps on how to keep your motivational fire burning.

ACTION STEPS

1. Remember your WHY

What is your reason for picking up this book? Are you feeling uncomfortable in your body? Are you done with not owning your natural glow? With feeling not-sexy in those gorgeous bathers or skinny jeans? Have you had enough of all the brain fog and overall grogginess from morning to evening? Have you decided you want to be back in control and not have your hormones ruling your life? Are your stress levels through the roof and you are longing to find your old patient, peaceful self again? Is your back killing you and your irregular sleep patterns are turning you into someone you don't want to be? If your why is about how you look or how much you weigh, you may struggle to keep your motivation. But, if your why is about how you want to feel and what you want to be able to do, then you have a powerful idea that you can anchor yourself to each day.

2. Don't go all out

Please don't blow up your motivation (and muscles) with a punishing, high-intensity burn. Instead, settle for one little step at a time which you commit to doing continuously. When your goal is to transition from a TV-watching potato coach to a strong, new, super fit version of yourself, it will best happen through incremental growth. I know it can be so very tempting to go all out and go from no training to 3-4 power sessions a week. After all, you want to see some results and you want them FAST. However, going about the new fit YOU in this very intense way will deny yourself the possibility to ease into and fall in love with your new lifestyle. Instead, you are putting your entire self in total shock-mode. You will probably end up dreading your next session and will find excuses to avoid this kind of torture ever again.

By throwing yourself into your transformation journey head over heels and at an insane speed, you totally run the risk that you are actually overtaxing yourself in a way that is neither sustainable nor particularly kind. The result is that you run out of steam pretty quickly. What's worse: once you realise you can simply not keep up with your crazy tempo, you will start feeling like a total loser too. Negative self-talk kicks in, which makes everything worse. You start doubting yourself and your comfy couch has never been more tempting. You push yourself into total defeat.

So, if you are in this wonder-licious new lifestyle for the long run, the answer lies in gifting your body, mind, and soul with progressive forms of movement in a slow and kind manner but CONTINUOUSLY. Wonder Woman—once you start, don't stop ever again!!!

3. Lose your inner perfectionist

Stay flexible and real. I am sorry I have to break it to you and bring you down from the clouds, but PERFECT does NOT EXIST. Trying to be perfect and doing everything 100% is another sure way to run straight into the I-can't-do-this-at-all wall. Trust me, I know what I am talking about. I am still a work in progress when it comes to letting go of my inner perfectionist, but the more I do, the bigger my wonderful world becomes. Not unlike going "all-out," you are putting yourself under enormous strain and pressure when your aim is total perfection, whether in this endeavour or in life in general.

When your goal is "perfect," you accomplish two things.

1. You make a lot of room for procrastination instead of tapping into your true strength of action.

2. You set yourself up for failure by having expectations of yourself that are far too high.

To find the success you want by this course of transformation you will need to embrace a good-enough mindset. Doing the work anyway, even if it might be beautifully imperfect, will take you so much further than putting things off and waiting for them or YOU to be more ready. Don't miss this wave of wanting to change because of something that is unachievable anyway. YOU ARE ENOUGH. You have always been enough and YOU ARE, NOW. Those magic words of GOOD ENOUGH will fast-forward you to where you want to be. Perfect will not. Going into your journey with the right mindset and expectations is more than a great foundation for turning those ambitions of yours into awesome feel-good reality.

4. Measure your success wisely

Measuring the success of your health goals is important. However, it is essential not to fall into the self-destructive, my-progress-and-self-worth-is-attached-to-how-much-I-weigh trap.

Transforming your life into wholesome healthfulness is all about nurturing your beautiful self with your best ability in any given moment. This means that using the scale to measure your progress is usually counter-productive. The scale can't measure your improved health, strength, fitness, or glow. It can't weigh the changes in body composition nor the deep satisfaction you feel when your endorphins are flowing.

Those misleading numbers on the scale do not show anything that is real about YOU. The scale is a tool that measures only a physical relationship with earth's gravity. So, how about evaluating your healthful victories using more empowering and reliable measures? Touch base with your gorgeous self and ask yourself: Do I feel more energetic and less tired? Has my skin cleared up? Do I look younger? Do people notice my changes so much that they stop to comment that I look amazing or to ask what is so intriguingly different about me? Have my aches and pains lifted? Do I have fewer colds? Do my clothes fit better (or do I need to buy clothes in smaller sizes so that I can wear right-fitting clothes?) Do I feel sexier and more fulfilled? How is my mental focus? Am I sleeping better? Have I lost my desire to overeat? What happened to the cravings that used to seem so important? Do I love feeling healthy?

5. Don't compare yourself to others—ever

"Comparison is the thief of joy," said Teddy Roosevelt, and it is the fastest way of killing all your positive I-can-do-this energy. Comparative thinking is crazy-making. You would never compare peas to beans and argue that peas are a more worthy vegetable. Of course, these amazing whole foods are both awesome and different. Obviously, they each offer their incredible gifts by being exactly what they're made to be. It is nonsense to compare them. Don't do it to yourself, either. What works for your best friend or work colleague might be the very thing that is wrong for you.

We are all different. It is therefore vitally important for your success that you adapt your new healthy-licious life to your liking, desires, wants, needs, character, fitness level, family situation, work-life, biological background, etc. You are truly like no one else in this whole wide wonderful world—indeed, there is no one like you in the whole wide expanse of the universe. You deserve for your journey to be wholly yours, independent of anyone else's path. I am calling upon your gorgeous, intuitive self to map out a plan that keeps you well encouraged all along the way.

If you hate running, trying to convince yourself that becoming an avid daily runner will give you your neighbour's great results—it just won't work. If you are 45 years of age and new to the gym, your training routine will look very different from your 30-year-old neighbour who has been a gym junkie her whole life. Do you get the individualised picture? Okay, before you commit to your new action plan, make sure it takes all your little quirks into account, everything that makes YOU gorgeously you. The more detailed you can draw this new lifestyle picture of yours, the better and more quickly you will see those results you are after.

6. Visualise your new self in the clearest detail possible

What can you do with a body that is fit, light, and strong? Where can you go? With whom? When? How do you feel? How do you dress? What do you look like? How do health and strength change your life? How does it empower you? What new activities can you explore? Envision every positive, empowering sensation as vividly as possible. Tap into them every time you can feel any doubt about your new journey creeping in on you. Bring them to life in your whole being every time you are running the risk of cancelling on yourself.

7. Look your glow in the eye

When was it that you felt your most wonderful, gorgeous, vibrant and fulfilled self? What was so different about you then? If you are a very visual person like I am, it might empower you to look this version of the beautiful YOU deeply in the eye as often as you can. You are already enough, today, just as you are AND you also deserve to remember and to remind yourself how much radiance you actually have inside yourself. This natural glow wants to be unleashed again. It is within you. It has always been there, but life got challenging somewhere along the way and you unlearned to nurture your sparkle. You unlearned to take those steps that bring you back to being this true goddess. It is time to look her in the eye again. Stick a picture of the glowing YOU, the one where you still believed in yourself, to your bathroom mirror to remind you who it truly is you are uncovering again.

8. Hold yourself accountable

Share your transformational journey with as many people as possible. The more you include your friends, family, and work colleagues in your wonderful plans, the better. I know how vulnerable this may make you feel—especially when self-doubt makes you question whether you can sustain this new, healthy, loving-movement lifestyle. Trust me, though—telling your world (especially your inner circle) about your goals has super-powers. It creates an energy that is undeniable and you are less likely to let them down than yourself. I know it sounds crazy, but my experience tells me this is very true. Having a little fan club of your very own and a personal cheerleader by your side is super powerful. It becomes so much harder to ditch the workout when you know you will be reporting this to someone who totally and utterly believes in you and your amazing progress of change. You will see. It is so much harder to let your friends down than yourself. At least in the beginning of your journey. So, while you might not be able to do this for yourself, yet...do it for them.

9. Allow soulful words to carry you through

Every day or at the very least, once per week, choose a new, meaningful mantra which you will keep repeating to yourself whenever you feel self-doubt creeping in on you. Pick a phrase, quote or sentence which truly empowers you and speaks straight to your soul. Repeat it to yourself upon waking up, in the shower, while you are eating, brushing your teeth, while you are driving, during your work breaks, while you go shopping, preparing dinner, doing the washing...as often as you need to hear those words to help you through your inner storm of insecurities. Allow your mantra to build a bridge of confidence and trust in your process until you can own it and fully believe in it yourself.

10. What role model do you choose to be?

Remind yourself of who is watching you. Yes, those children of yours have their eyes and ears everywhere. It is super scary, but they truly are like little sponges. They soak up everything you do (and don't do!). They store within themselves everything they see as being their ideal world. You, as their parent, are their total hero. They perceive you as the one who has all the answers, who knows how to get things right and how to live their best life. What you do and say is their raw blueprint as they move forward in creating their own life. In those moments when your motivation is quivering, ask yourself whether you want your children to learn to get up and do it anyway or to come up with excuses why they should not. Trust me...they are watching and listening to all of YOU all of the time.

11. Focus your energy on what makes you strong

Train your thinking to see the awesome, feel-good, I-am-powerful feeling you have after you have been moving your body. Look at how you overcame your initial resistance to simply beginning and ponder over the radiant glow you feel after you have stretched, strengthened, and breathed love into your body. All this amazing exuberance and vitality is your winning ticket! Your past paradigm can never talk you out of this wonder-licious satisfaction, this incredible strength, this supercharged mind, one workout at a time. The yummy-licious trust you are re-discovering in your own capacity will have you shouting to your friends, "I love it! I love ME!"

12. Enjoy the ride

Embrace every single moment of your journey; cast aside judgement over the length of it and be in gratitude for the gift of each moment. Dive into this process so deeply that you become it. Imagine that you have gone for a run or started your training session, but your thoughts are centred only on the time you are spending or the distance you must cover. These ideas rob you of enjoying every step or move you make. Your transformation journey is not different. Negative thoughts demotivate you from your purpose. I know it because I have been there. It is awful to tell yourself that you are unfit, slow, and weak. It is drudgery to wonder if you will ever go far enough, well enough to even make a difference. What is heavy becomes heavier. However, if you will simply relax into the moment and centre your attention on how your body is changing with every single step, you will love the process so much that you will not even notice how steep your climb is. More than this: you will grow wings to fly over those rocky bits on your way.

OBSTACLE 2: A BIG DOSE OF SELF-SABOTAGE IS RUSHING IN

ACTION STEPS TO FIGHT OFF THE SELF-MANIPULATIVE YOU:

1. Don't let your mind bully you

Be clear with yourself about what is happening right now inside your mind. It is playing tricks on you to keep you where you are right now. In your 'happy,' 'safe,' nothing-will-ever-move-forward zone. Don't ever let your mind boss you around. Have you ever sat down with the ambition to meditate in the spaces of your hectic life, to clear your thoughts, reduce stress, and come back to your heart, only to then sit there being totally torn apart by unkind, intrusive thoughts interrupting the Zen you are trying to generate? Does your meditation practise look more like:

"I don't have time to do this..."
"Breathe, darling, breathe..."
"Ohhhhkay... feeling bliss..."
"Shit! I have to email that client!"
"Easy there, Beautiful... breathing, feeling bliss..."

All of this, on a wash-rinse-repeat cycle of no-sanity and NOT bliss that it might seem totally funny if it was not so dead-on accurate. Looking at it from the outside, it is indeed very funny. In fact, this is the very MIND I am inviting you to see for yourself which can be doing this craziness to you.

2. You are not your emotion

Recognise that your fear is just an emotion, not reality. Imagine embracing your sabotaging-shoulder devil with a gentle hug. Then with the same care, and also great decisiveness, shake her off your shoulder and set yourself free. Wave at her or blow her a kiss and deliberately step into the other direction. I really love imagining my own self-sabotaging efforts, fears, and insecurities as little devils jumping onto my shoulders, tugging on my shirt, climbing up to my ears and whispering to me all my self-limiting beliefs and worries they can possibly think of. It makes it easier for me to point out to all the other parts of me that I am not those devils. I am in total control of what I do with those voices. Give it a try—see if this works for you just as beautifully.

3. Create a clear vision in line with your goal

Take the first step to making your dreams happen. Focus on your goal, making your vision of the healthy-licious YOU as clear as possible. You need to be able to see it and feel it to be able to make it your reality. One little word of warning: do not fall into the trap of limiting yourself here, though. Sometimes, especially for people who struggle to own their magnificence, it is so challenging to grasp all the magic that you are and may be about to uncover. So, while clearly imagining what you want, think big and stay open to the possibility that you are about to encounter a much more vibrant version of YOU than you ever could have believed was possible.

4. Replace your fear with positivity

Give the goal in your life more power and room than you give to your fear. Replace fear with self-compassion and hope by telling yourself the joyful truth your fear has never known. When your fear tries to persuade you that your efforts are futile and reminds you how many times you pointlessly failed, kindly remember that you are totally capable of doing this and that you are closer than you think to where you want to be. I believe the bigger the attempt of self-sabotage, the more powerful you actually are on this journey...the more amazing your results are going to be...the more glowing and wonderful, the outcome!!! The more positivity you nourish within yourself, the stronger you will be on taking the next step forward, leaving your fear way back behind you. "Hey, Fear—Sorry, not sorry!"

5. You are not your beliefs

Check in with your beliefs. Are they truly serving you or do they need an empowerment upgrade? Perhaps it is time to go on a discovery hunt within your precious self; look back at your life and get clear on where those beliefs stem from. Did you take on from a close family member the idea that you lack willpower or that you don't love healthy food? Were you labelled as someone who is not good at sports or who fails to see things through to their end? Did someone give you the idea that you are stuck in a big body or that you have no idea when to stop eating? Or did one of your parents show their love by treating you to sweet baked goodies or ice cream? Did you learn early on in your life that comfort has a sweet taste?

Now allow yourself to rediscover the innocent, health goddess you were before such comments or learnt behaviours hit hard your precious soul and twisted your beliefs. This is the true YOU. You are not your self-limiting belief(s). They are just a coat that is hanging over you, covering up the true you. Can you remember who you were without that coat? Did you love moving? Did you enjoy your precious body? Did you know exactly how to give yourself love when you needed it without relying on sweet treats? I invite you to, little by little, get rid of your coat and come back to owning your true, healthy-licious self again.

Weight Loss and Movement

It pains me to see women all over the globe thinking of exercise as something that will rectify their nutrition-poor diet. Exercise is not meant to punish your body for what you ate. Your body does not function like this. Losing weight through movement is not as simple as only upping your caloric output (that is, burning more calories through engaging in more movement). What they say is true: You cannot out-train a diet that is based on foods that do not nurture your body. So, let's drop once and for all the mindset which alienates a flourishing, mutual relationship between you and your precious physical self. Just to be clear, this does not mean that moving your body is not one of the most empowering ways to make your body transformation journey a total success—it's simply that movement is not about weight loss. Movement is about love and nurture, and while it can support your weight loss, it will not singlehandedly transform your body. Not as long as you do not give your diet a loving overhaul too, at least. But let's not jump ahead of ourselves, we'll explore more on this later.

WHY IS EXERCISE INEFFECTIVE AS A SOLE STRATEGY FOR WEIGHT LOSS?

The reason is pretty plain and simple. If your intended course is to continue to eat the same volume of the same food and drink that you consumed when you gained the extra weight, simply adding movement to your regimen will not magically cause this extra weight to fall off you. Yes, you might lose a little weight since you are burning more calories than before, but when I say "a little," I mean, a little. In addition, you are also very likely to increase your muscle tone, which is much more dense than fat and will generally translate into gaining weight. Being more active will also increase your appetite, naturally leading you to eating more, even if you are not aware of it. The sum effect is obviously that you will not make great progress in your weight-loss journey.

LET'S TALK ABOUT FAT-LOSS, THOUGH, AS OPPOSED TO JUST WEIGHT-LOSS

And here comes the great news: Increasing your movement and exercise level does give your body composition a wonderful make-over. Engaging in forms of cardiovascular or aerobic exercise will boost your body's ability to burn fat. Making a healthy strength routine fit into your empowered new life will stimulate your muscles to grow stronger and bigger. Your muscles are metabolically active tissue, meaning the more toned you are, the more calories you will be burning at rest. While a toned, strong body might not be necessarily also a light one, it will look amazingly sexy and be your best insurance policy to not pile those kilos onto your waist line whenever you overeat. In case this came out wrong: Obviously those toned muscles will not help you against overeating itself (that would be awesome!), but since muscle is metabolic active tissue, it helps you burn more calories. So, when you do happen to eat too much here and there, this will not show so quickly on your goddess body in the form of fat.

THERE ARE MORE REASONS TO CHOOSE FAT-LOSS OVER WEIGHT LOSS:

Weight loss does not necessarily spiral your health forward. What??? Yes, it is true. Because weight loss, particularly rapid weight loss, is most often due to a loss of water. Given that our bodies are more than sixty percent water (an adult body, that is), this loss is neither healthy nor transformative. It is not what you are striving for. Losing water weight will not enable you to live longer nor to fight heart disease, cancer, diabetes, or any number of chronic conditions that lower your quality of life. Not only that, weight loss that follows water loss often comes from losing precious muscle tissue. Losing muscle tissue brings its own load of adverse health conditions. Our resting metabolic rate slows down which means we burn fewer calories. Now diabetes, obesity and hormonal turmoil has just come a huge step closer. We are more prone to osteoporosis, osteoarthritis, and all those strength-related issues, including back pain. What is the most frustrating piece in all of this is that none of this weight loss has done a thing to reduce the unwanted fat that we hold in our beautiful bodies, especially the fat surrounding our precious organs. This fat is what makes us sick, causes heart attacks, and shortens our life span. We end up on a long list of pharmaceuticals to lower our blood pressure or fighting our levels of unhealthy cholesterol. You have taken on this transformation journey to win. You are in it to feel and look your best self again. You want to look and feel toned, strong, and sexy. You don't want to simply have a lower number on the scale—you want bone-deep strength, health, and beauty *that glows from the inside out.*

Did you know that a thin body is not necessarily healthier than a thick body? I am not arguing for you to be content living in a body that is too big for your frame or one that does not feel amazing. I am stating a simple truth that "thin does not automatically indicate health." This again comes down to body composition. If a body looks outwardly thin, but has a hidden load of visceral fat, then that body is just as prone to inflammations, gastric upset, and metabolic chaos. This condition is called "skinny obese" and may very well pose a greater health risk than for someone who is thick, simply because the threat is hidden and we are programmed in our western mindset to prefer thin bodies. People who are outwardly thin and inwardly obese may feel less inclined or pressured to pursue greater health if their physical condition is accepted as beautiful. These candidates are not only less likely to put on their athletic shoes and get sweaty, they are also less likely to have anyone suggest that they should.

ON A PSYCHOLOGICAL LEVEL, WEIGHT LOSS CAN BE SO DESTRUCTIVE WHILE FAT LOSS HAS UPLIFTING SUPER-POWERS

When we focus on weight loss as our ultimate goal, without regard to how we accomplish that loss, we are running the bitter risk of focusing on all the wrong things and for all the wrong reasons. We pay attention to the numbers on the scale, rather than making our well-being our top priority. We obsess about numbers with complete disregard to the fact that the scale cannot measure health nor increase our self-worth. We take comfort in the illusion of control offered by the scale and try to ignore, outwit, or silence our body's voice. We credit the scale for knowing more about our body than our body knows about itself. The scale cannot know your body from mine; it does not know whether you have bones that are more dense or whether your body has more muscle tone; it cannot tell us what our bodies know, which is this: We are beautiful and capable souls with an innate ability to heal, grow, and thrive.

Our bodies know what we need to transform and become to be the best, most healthy form we can be. Our bodies await only our listening to the intuitive powers of transformation that live within us.

More often than not, when you step on the scale you think you are measuring progress, but instead, you are actually doing harm. You are hurting your heart and your soul. You are threatening your self-confidence. You are feeding the temptation to demonize your body for being stubborn and ill-suited for beauty and life. Instead of concentrating your thoughts on how your body CAN feel, you are devolving into a world of punishment and self-loathing negativity. You are giving permission to the numbers displayed on a simple machine to define your worth and your capacity for a stunningly beautiful life. The scale is not your friend.

On the other hand, when you measure your success by your inch-by-inch, step-by-step growth in becoming a healthier, stronger version of yourself, you are beginning a practise of self-nurture, self-compassion, and self-love. Your body will begin to glow with the light of one who is well loved, and while the scale may be slow to mirror such glow, your body will warm and shine with truth. You will come to crave natural, whole food. You will feel powerful in the knowledge and truth of yourself, whispered so softly and sweetly from your heart and soul. Your body will willingly surrender all that does not serve its vitality when it feels the safety of your respect, the reverence of your gratitude, and kind and loving energy of your heart. You will feel sexy and carry yourself with undeniably beautiful confidence. Your energy will be positive and uplifted. Your mind-body connection will only deepen. You will begin living a life of wisdom, ever forward-moving and ever calmly assured that you are in a beautiful love affair with the divine glory you carry within. You will become masterful in this peaceful partnership with your body, always working together for your best life.

This is possible for you if fat loss happens sensibly. Again, this is not about numbers and percentages. This isn't about obsessing about numbers fitting into a column on a BMI chart. This is about allowing yourself to become your healthiest, most glowing version of yourself. You deserve to know that for most women, aged 20-60 years, healthy body fat ranges between 21-35%. Of course, in younger women there is naturally a lower level of fat, and this is simply due to the biological fact that we lose muscle mass as we age. This is why it is truly so important to fall in love with strengthening your precious muscles and bones. Always remember to honour YOUR body and YOUR shape; the fat loss that matters is the disease and inflammation inducing belly fat.

USE MOVEMENT TO MAKE YOUR HEALTHY FAT-LOSS HAPPEN

The most effective way to nurture your body with all three forms of movement is to do them *continuously in small, bite-sized time slots*. It is the day-by-day, week-by-week, month-by-month consistency that will make all the difference to your healthy-licious self. If you can build a routine and come back to a particular movement around the same time each day and each week, your body will eventually start burning fat at that time, simply in anticipation of your workout. Is that not incredible? Our bodies are insanely amazing!

Try this: If you are new to your healthy-licious life, commit to thirty minutes each day of low to moderate cardiovascular exercise. If you are more experienced, find a simple upgrade to your already-established healthy movement practise. It may be more time or it may be increased intensity (choose one or the other, not both).

In addition:

Try and commit one to three times each week to strength train. Twenty minutes is totally enough, or even small tabata training sets of 4 minutes (which are high intensity interval training workouts that are super effective in a short amount of time), repeated two or three times. If you are just beginning this practise, start with one. Increase it each week[3].

Remember not to do two consecutive days of working the same muscle groups. Alternate muscle groups day by day or rest a day in between. The exception is your core—you can work your core muscles daily if it feels right in your body.

In addition, to improve flexibility:

Try to commit to 1-3 times weekly of lengthening stretches or yoga sessions—ten to twenty minutes can be sufficient and make huge changes to your entire well-being. If you are newly adding flexibility training to your healthy-licious movement practise, begin with one session and gradually increase to two or three sessions each week, if time allows. If you are not a big fan of yoga, you can add more extensive stretches right after your cardio and strength workouts. Remember—find your way around it and make it fit into your busy lifestyle.

---

3 **Note** Doing two strength workouts per week is so much easier than doing a single one. Doing one almost feels like restarting each time (which isn't true), but when you are doing more strength sessions per week, your body seems to stay more in the flow.

LET'S PLAY

EMPOWERING ALL BODY WORKOUT
TO IGNITE YOUR MAGIC GLOW

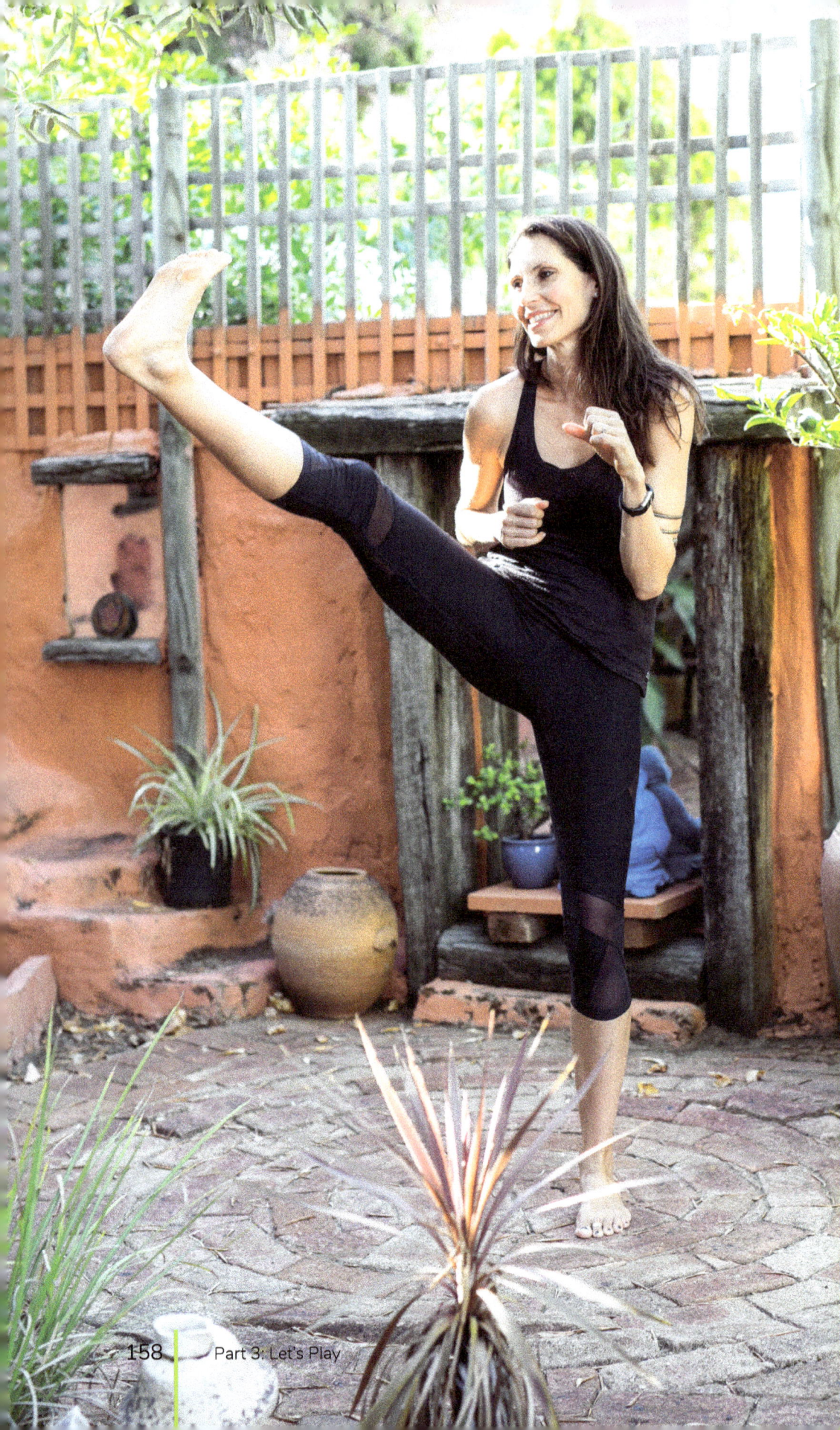

My exercise philosophy is that it is essential to make my workout as efficient as possible. My life is crazy-busy, so it is a total treat for me and my clients to work as many muscle groups as possible in one exercise. This allows your blood flow to rush from one end of your body to the next, working hard every precious part of your physical self. This not only increases your heart rate and fat burn, but also empowers you with good core strength. Talking about core strength: In my moving world, there is no exercise that does not also strengthen my core. With a strong core, you can do anything!

Not only that, when you coordinate different movements to different parts of your body, you are giving your brain a fabu-licious workout too. This can prevent dementia and other age-related issues. Prevention is better than a cure and it is never too early to start.

I invite you to use YOUR precious time as effectively as I do. Are you ready to come and play with me? Let's do this!

Here is one of my favourite exercise routines for you to play around and have fun with at home:

What you need:

1. YOU, you gorgeous woman!

2. Two hand towels (or, if training on carpet, two paper plates) or sliders

3. If you have dumbbells it is a plus, but you can do this routine also with water bottles or without using any added resistance and simply using your own body weight.

4. A timer. Set it for eight rounds of 25 seconds on and ten seconds off (Tabata training)

Enjoy!

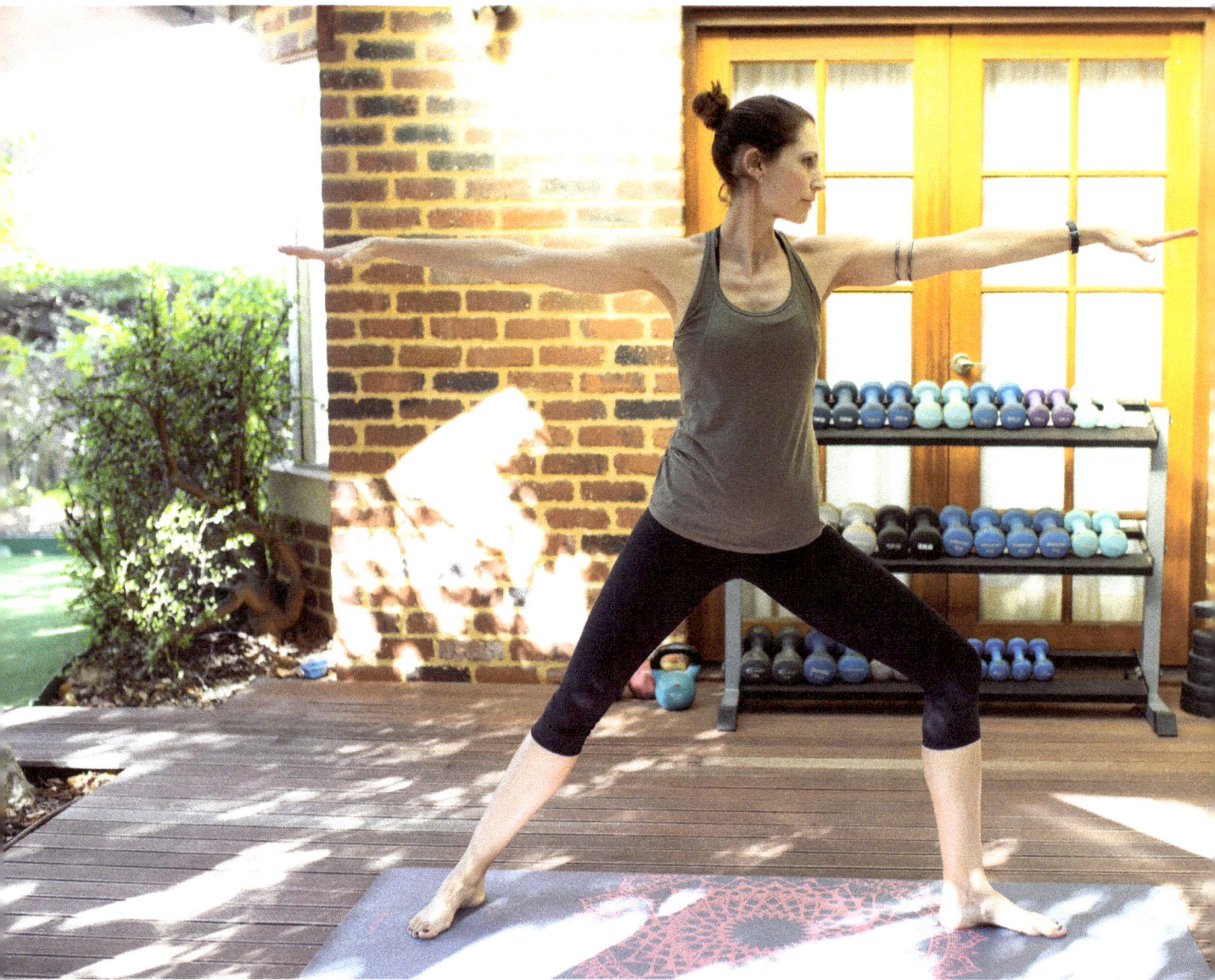

EXERCISES

A Exercise: Rock Your Body

1. Start in pike push-up position and perform 1 pike push-up, bending your arms.

2. Jump your legs into your hands, lifting your hands off the ground so you will land in a low squat.

3. Landing in a low squat, bring your arms backwards to perform a triceps kick-back with your arms. Pay attention to keep your knees in line with your middle toe and behind your toes. This works your shoulders, upper back, quads, glutes, triceps, biceps and core.

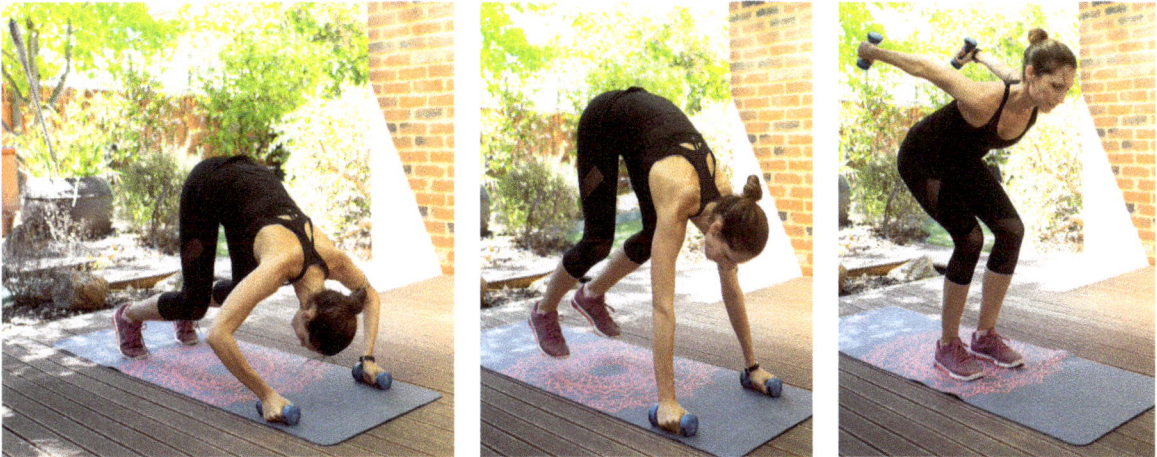

B Exercise: Strong Core Hello

1. Start lying with your back flat on the ground and your arms outstretched overhead. Lift your upper back off the ground, driving your navel into the spine.

2. Lift your upper body off the ground, keeping a long spine, while lifting one of your outstretched legs then bringing that leg towards your head.

3. Bend your leg, bringing the knees to the chest and reach towards your heel. Reset and start with move 1 again, followed by move 2 and repeat move 3 on the other side. This works your core and lower abs.

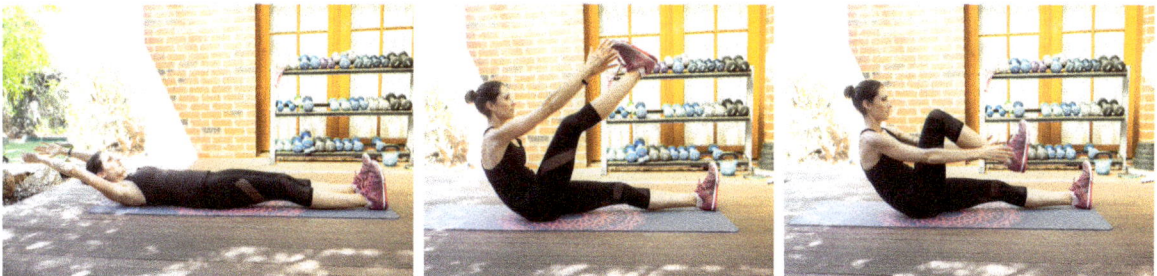

C Exercise: Totally Not Creepy Crawlers

1. Start in a normal push-up position and perform 1 push-up on toes or on knees.

2. Slide legs wide on sliders or towels and perform a wide legged push-up.

3. Slide 1 leg forward and same side arm forward and perform lizard push-up. Reset and start with move 1 again, followed by move 2, then repeat on the other side. This works your chest, shoulder, arm and core muscles.

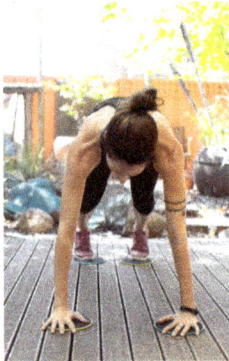

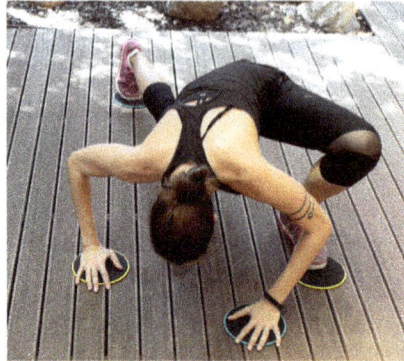

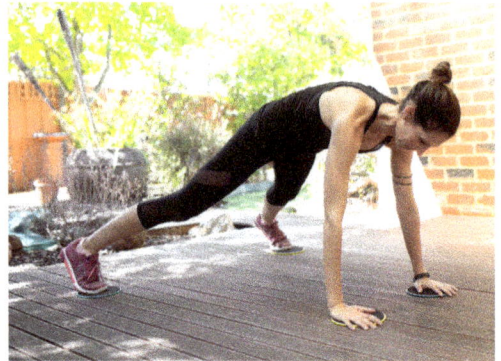

D Exercise: Sexy Back

1. Start with your belly lying flat on the ground, weights in hand, then lift your upper and lower body as high as you can, lifting your arms behind your body as high as you can. Keep your neck neutral.

2. Reverse your arm movement, lower your legs and upper body and lift yourself up in one straight line into a plank position.

3. Bring one of your knees to your chest, rounding your upper body. Reset and start with move 1 again, followed by move 2 and repeat move 3 on the other side. This works your core, lower and upper back, and triceps muscles.

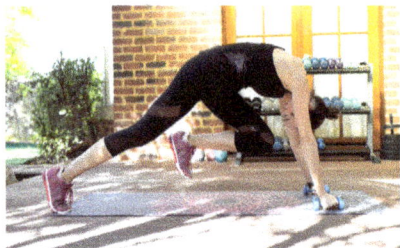

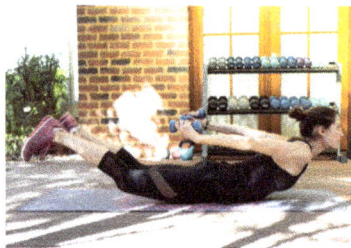

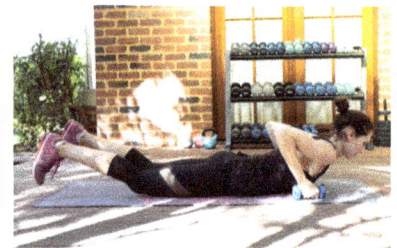

E Exercise: Goddess Legs, Glutes and Arms

1. From standing, slide 1 leg back into lunge position while bending arms from overhead to just above your head. Pay attention to keep your knee in line with your middle toe and your knee behind your toes. Try to create a 90° angle with your foot, thigh and torso.

2. Slide the leg back into squat position, keeping legs bent and hips low, while performing a biceps curl.

3. Keeping hips low, slide the opposite leg back into lunge position, bringing the arms overhead again and curling behind the neck. This works all of your leg muscles, glutes, arms, shoulders and core.

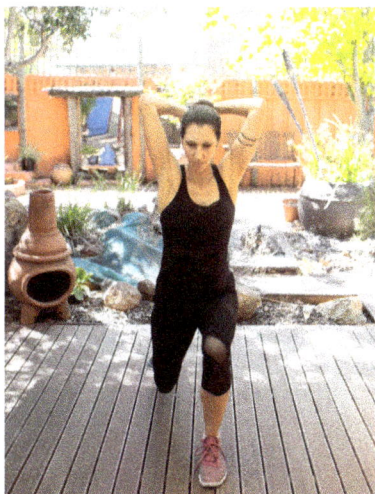

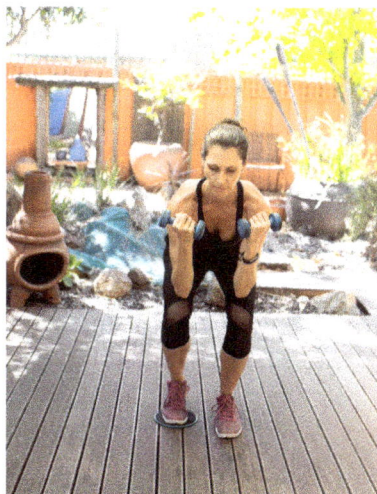

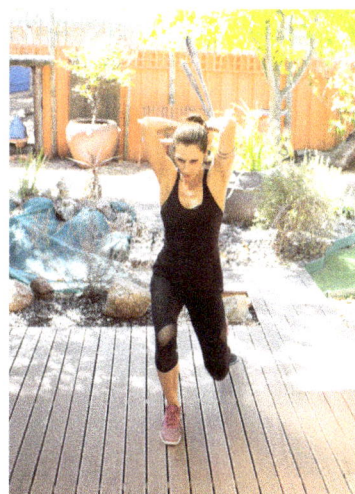

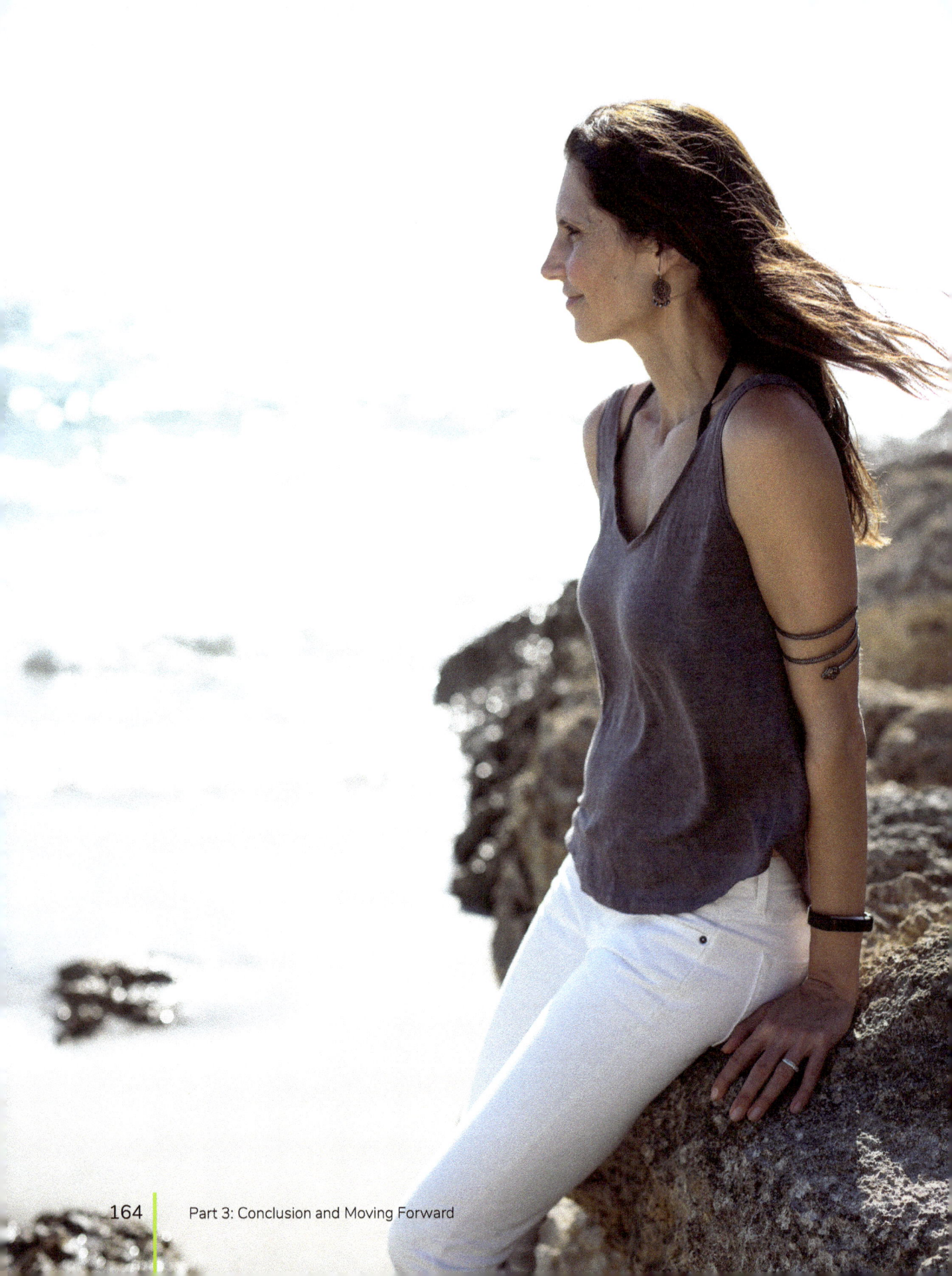

Part 3: Conclusion and Moving Forward

Conclusion and Moving Forward

Yay ... you made it through the entire book!!! Well done!!!

Maybe you feel a little overwhelmed now having been introduced to so many insights and so much information. Maybe all of this seems a lot at first glance and therefore, a little bit overwhelming. I have no doubt, though, that YOU have totally got this!!! You picked up this book for a reason! You are so ready to dive in head first and embark on this amazing journey towards the happiest, most glowing, vibrant YOU! You are done not giving your beautiful body, mind, and soul what it deserves and needs! You are so ready to love and nurture yourself the healthy-licious way. You have had enough of beating yourself up with negative self-talk, elusive diets, and painful exercises. YOU know that you are here to live your best life full of tender self-compassion and care!!! And this is exactly what you are about to do!!!

Remember to take it one action step at a time. Keep in mind that it's all a wild dance of two steps forward and one step back. Smile at yourself often—especially on those days when things feel a little harder or more stuck!!! Ask yourself on those days whether you are still nourishing all of you with the utmost self-respect towards yourself. Are you attentively listening to all the subtle messages your body is giving you? Are you taking care of your soul and heart? Then you are doing fantastically well!!! Think of my many falls. They might not have been pretty at the time but they brought me to where I am now and made me so much stronger and more powerful. Enjoy this journey, it is truly amazing. Feel free to share with me how your individual dance looks and feels. I would love to hear from you!!! Also, know that I have got your back always!!!

Trust that everything is exactly happening when and the way it is meant to be—you are doing just fine!!!! So, it's over to you, Gorgeous. Put a stunning smile on your face first and then take your leap of faith! You were born to feel wonderful in your skin—nothing less. Let's make sure YOU do!!!!!!!!

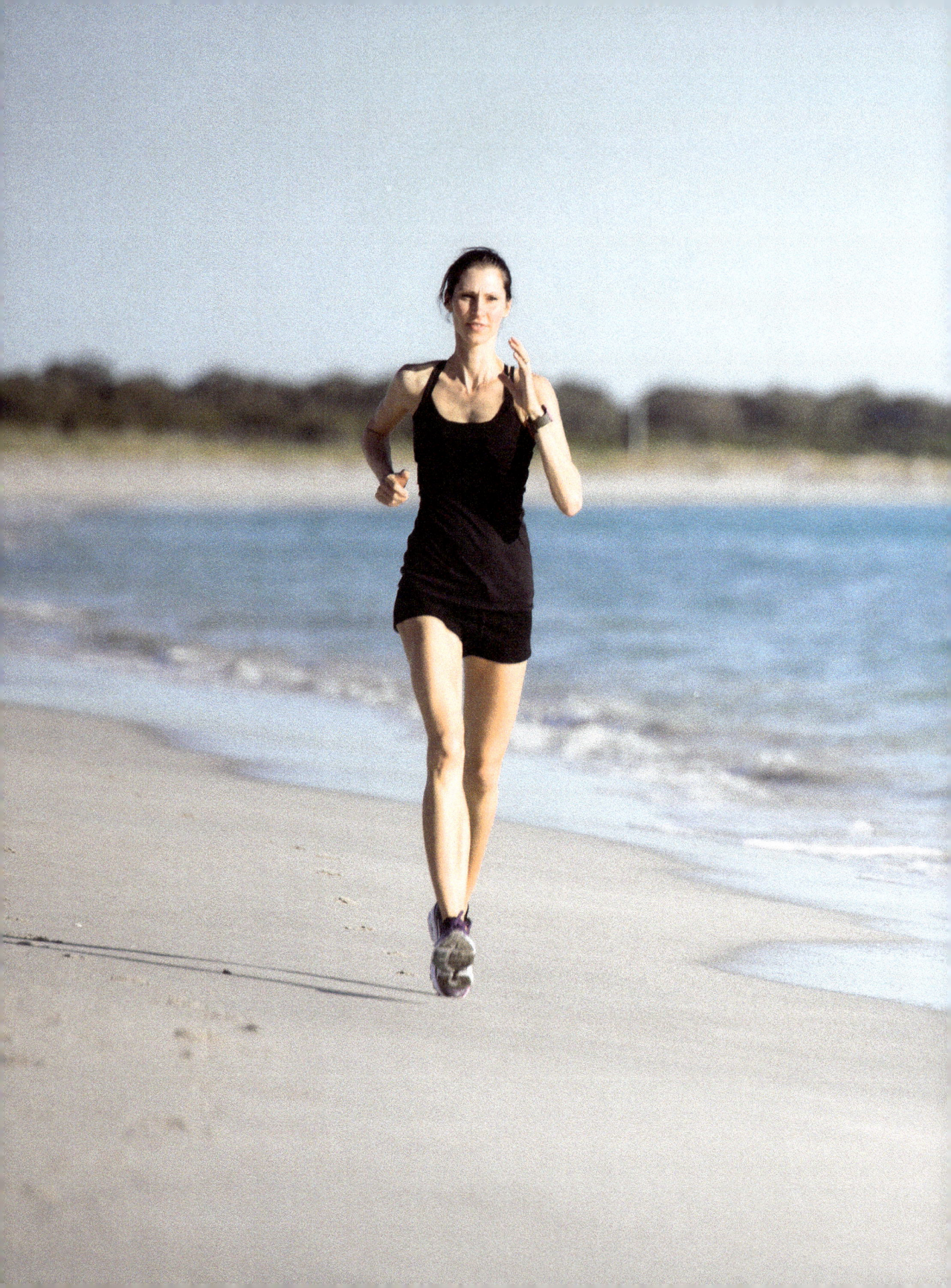

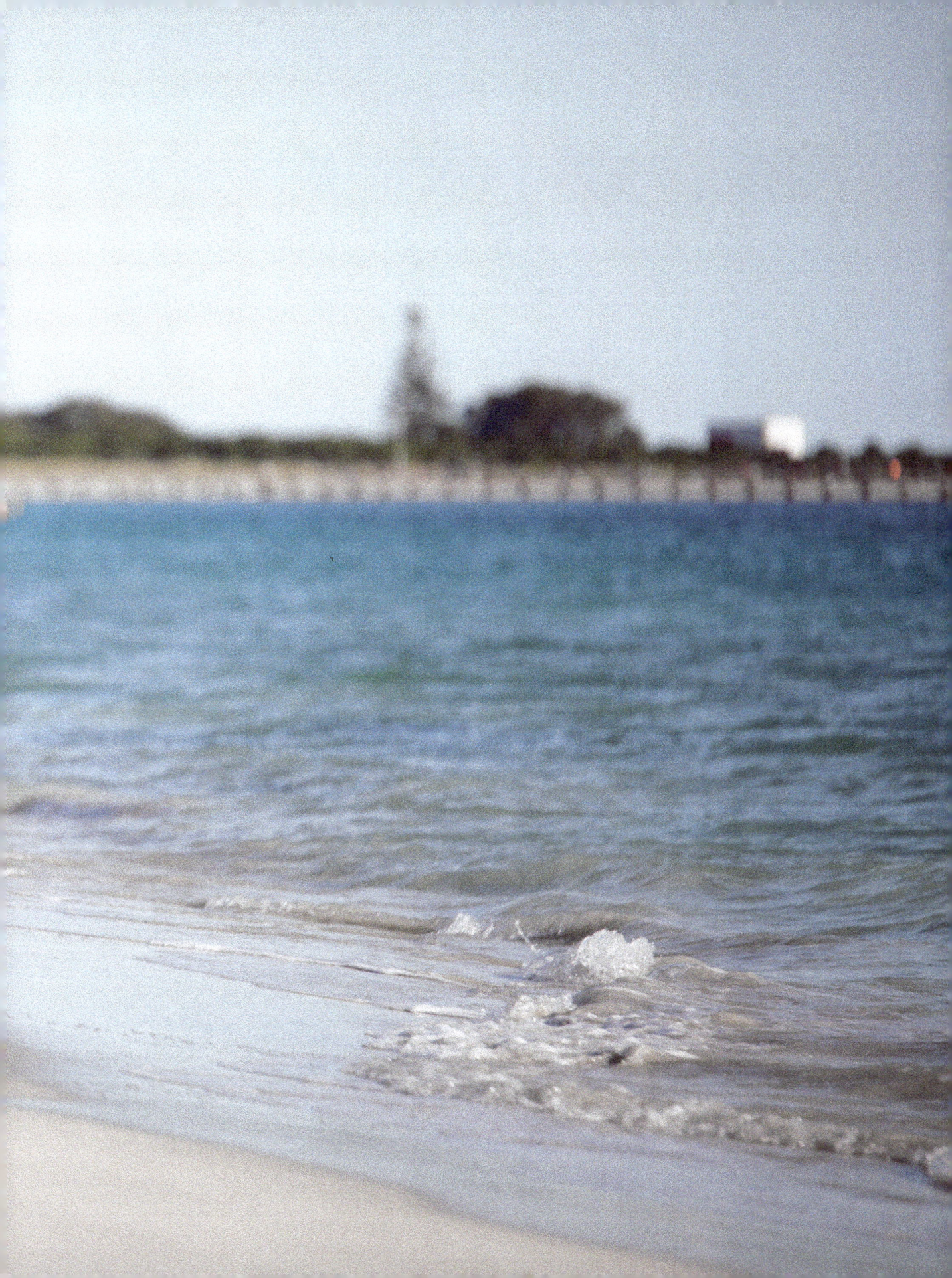

Reference List

Part 1:

Cosgrove, F. 2007, *Coach yourself to wellness living the intentional life*, 1st edn, Messenger Publishing, Australia.

Rosenthal, J. 2011, *Integrative nutrition feed your hunger for health & happiness*, 3rd edn, Greenleaf Book, New York.

Prochaska, J. O., Redding, C. A., Revers, K. E. (2015). 'The transtheoretical model and stages of change', in Glanz, K., Rimer, B. K., Visvanath, K. (ed.) *Health Behaviour: Theory, Research and Practice*. San Francisco C.A., pp.125-148.

Seravalle, G., Mancia, G., Grassi, G. 2018 20:74. 'Sympathetic nervous system, sleep, and hypertension', *Current Hypertension Reports*, vol. 20, issue 74, https://doi.org/10.1007/s11906-018-0874-y

Danisi, J., Fernandez-Mendoza J., Vgontzas, A. N., Bixler, O. E. 2019, 'The behavioral, molecular, pharmacological, and clinical basis of the sleep-wake cycle', *Science Direct*, pp. 123-142, https://doi.org/10.1016/B978-0-12-816430-3.00007-5

Yaribeygi, H., Panahi, Y., Sahraei, H., Johnston, T. P. Sahebkar, A. 2017, 'The impact of stress on body function: a review', *Excli Journal*, vol. 16, pp. 1057-1072, 10.17179/excli2017-480

Racz, B., Duskova, M., Starka, L., Hainer, V., Kunesova, M 2018, 'Links between the circadian rhythm, obesity and the microbiome', *Physiological Research*, vol. 67, issue 3, pp. 409-420, https://www.biomed.cas.cz/physiolres/pdf/67/67_S409.pdf

Stavrou, V., Bardaka, F., Karetsi, E., Daniil, Z., Gourgoulianis, K. I. 2018, 'Brief Review: Ergospirometry in patients with obstructive sleep apnea syndrome,' *Pathergasiology & Psychology*, vol. 7, p. 191, https://doi.org/10.3390/jcm7080191

Murawski, B., Wade, L., Plotnikoff, R. C., Lubans, D. R., Duncan, M. J. 2018, 'A systematic review and meta-analysis of cognitive and behavioural interventions to improve sleep health in adults without sleep disorders', *Sleep Medicine Reviews*, vol. 40, pp. 160-169, https://doi.org/10.1016/j.smrv.2017.12.003Get rights and content

Lederle, Dr K 2018, *Sleep sense*, Exisle Publishing, Chatswood, NSW, Australia.

Yaribeygi, H., Panahi, Y., Sahraei, H., Johnston, T. P., Sahebkar, A. 2017, 'The impact of stress on body function: a review,' *Excli Journal Experimental and Clinical Services*, vol. 16, pp. 1057-1072, 10.17179/excli2017-480

Everly, Jr GS, Lating, JM, Jeffrey M. 1989, *A clinical guide to the treatment of the human stress response*, 4th edn, Springer, New York, USA.

Chu, L-Ch. 2010, 'The benefits of meditation via-a-vis emotional intelligence, perceived stress and negative mental health', *Stress & Health*, vol. 26, issue 2, pp. 169-180, https://doi.org/10.1002/smi.1289

Horowitz, S. 2010, 'Health benefits of meditation: what the newest research shows', *Alternative and Complementary Therapies*, vol. 16, issue 4, https://doi.org/10.1089/act.2010.16402

Davis, D. M., & Hayes, J. A. (2011). What are the benefits of mindfulness? A practice review of psychotherapy-related research', *Psychotherapy*, 48, issue 2, pp. 198-208. http://dx.doi.org/10.1037/a0022062

Ross, A., Thomas, S. 2010, 'The health benefits of yoga and exercise: a review of comparison studies', The Journal of Alternative and Complementary Medicine, vol 16, issue 1, http://doi.org/10.1089/acm.2009.0044

Cowen, V. S., Adams, T. B. 2005, 'Physical and perceptual benefits of yoga asana practice: results of a pilot study', *Journal of Bodywork and Movement Therapies*, vol. 9, issue 3, pp. 211-219, https://doi.org/10.1016/j.jbmt.2004.08.001

Monk-Turner, E. 2003, 'The benefits of meditation: experimental findings', *The Social Science Journal*, vol. 40, issue 3, pp. 465-470, https://doi.org/10.1016/S0362-3319(03)00043-0

Shonin, E., Van Gordon, W., Griffiths, M. D. 2013, 'Meditation as medication: are attitudes changing?', *British Journal of General Practice*, vol. 63, issue 617, p. 654, https://doi.org/10.3399/bjgp13X675520

Tang, Y.-Y., Ma, Y., Wang, J., Fan, Y., Feng, S., Lu, Q., Yu, Q., Sui, D., Rothbart, M. K., Fan, M. Posner, M. I. 2007, 'Short-term meditation training improves attention and self-regulation', *Proceedings of the National Academy of Sciences of the United States of America*, vol. 104, issue 43, pp. 17152-17156, https://doi.org/10.1073/pnas.0707678104

Part 2:

Rolfes, S.R., Pinna, K., Whitney, E. 2009, *Understanding normal and clinical nutrition*, 8th edn, Wadsworth Cengage Learning, Belmont, CA.

Whitney, E., Rolfes, S. R. 2018, *Understanding Nutrition*, 15th edn, Cengage, Boston, MA.

Porth, C. M., Matfin, G. 2009, *Pathophysiology Concepts of altered health states*, 8th edn, Lippincott-Raven, Philadelphia.

Cooper, L. 2016, *Accredited certificate of nutrition*, 7th edn, Cadence Health, Sydney.

Slavin, J. 2007, 'Why whole grains are protective: biological mechanisms', *Proceedings of The Nutrition Society*, vol. 62, issue 1, pp. 129-134, https://doi.org/10.1079/PNS2002221

Vasey, C. 2006, *The acid-alkaline diet for optimum health: restore your health by creating pH balance in your diet*, 2nd edn, Healing Arts Press, Rochester, VT.

Toomath, R. 2016, *Why diets and exercise don't work – and what does*, 1st edn, Auckland University Press, Auckland.

Applebaum, M. 2008, 'Why diets fail – expert diet advice as a cause of diet failure', *American Psychologist*, vol. 63, issue 3, pp. 200-202, https://psycnet.apa.org/buy/2008-03389-008

Buchanan, K., Sheffield, J. 2015, 'Why do diets fail? An exploration of dieters' experiences using thematic analyis', *Journal of Health Psychology*, vol. 22, issue 7, 2017, https://doi.org/10.1177%2F1359105315618000

Wanders, A. J., van den Borne, J. J. G. C., de Graaf, C., Hulshof, T., Jonathan, M. C., Kristinsen, M., Mars, M., Schols, H. A., Freskens, E. J. M. 2011, 'Effects of dietary fibre on subjective appetite, energy intake and body weight: a systematic review of randomized controlled trials', Obesity Reviews, vol. 12, issue 9, pp.724-739, https://doi.org/10.1111/j.1467-789X.2011.00895.x

Kwok, A., Dordevic, A. L., Paton, G., Page, M. J. 2019, 'Effect of alcohol consumption on food energy intake: a systematic review and meta-analysis', British Journal of Nutrition, vol, 121, issue 5, pp. 481-495, https://doi.org/10.1017/S0007114518003677

Dunn, C., Haubenreiser, M., Johnson, M., Nordby, K. Aggarwal, S., Myer. S., Thomas, C. 2018, 'Mindfulness approaches and weight loss, weight maintenance, and weight regain', Current Obesity Reports, vol. 7, issue 1, pp. 37-49, https://link.springer.com/article/10.1007/s13679-018-0299-6#citeas

Cooper, L., 2014, Change the Way You Eat: The Psychology of Food, 1st edn, Exisle Publishing, Auckland.

Cosgrove, F. 2007, Coach yourself to wellness living the intentional life, 1st edn, Messenger Publishing, Australia.

Tortora, G. J., Derrickson, B. 2009, Principles of anatomy and physiology, 12th edn, Wiley, USA.

Avena, N. M., Talbott, J. R. 2014, Why diets fail (because you're addicted to sugar): science explains how to end cravings, lose weight, and get healthy, 1st edn, Ten Speed Press, New York.

Avena, N. M., Rada P., Hoebel, B. G. 2008, 'Evidence for sugar addiction: behavioural and neurochemical effects of intermittent, excessive sugar intake', Neuroscience & Biobehavioral Reviews, vol. 31, issue 1, pp. 20-39, https://doi.org/10.1016/j.neubiorev.2007.04.019

Malik, V.S., Schulze M. B, Hu F. B. 2006, 'Intake of sugar-sweetened beverages and weight gain: a systematic review', The American Journal of Clinical Nutrition, vol. 84, issue 2, pp. 274-288, https://doi.org/10.1093/ajcn/84.2.274

Lowe, M. R., Butryn, M. L. 2007, 'Hedonic hunger: a new dimension of appetite?', Physiology & Behaviour, vol. 91, issue 4, pp.432-439, https://doi.org/10.1016/j.physbeh.2007.04.006

Gameau, D. & Z. 2016, That sugar guide, 1st edn, Pan Macmillan, Sydney, Australia.

Mirtschink, P., Jang, C., Arany, Z., Krek, W. 2018, 'Fructose metabolism, cardiometabolic risk and the epidemic of coronary artery disease', European Heart Journal, vol. 39, issue 26, pp. 2497-2505, https://doi.org/10.1093/eurheartj/ehx518

Glenville, M. 2006, Fat around the middle, 1st edn, Kyle Cathie, London.

Murphy, J. 2011, The power of your subconscious mind, Matino Publishing, Mansfield Centre, CT.

Steel, D., Kemps, E., Tiggemann, M. 2006, 'Effects of hunger and visio-spatial interference on imagery-induced food cravings', Appetite, vol. 46, issue 1, pp. 36-40, https://doi.org/10.1016/j.appet.2005.11.001

Hill, A. J., Weaver, C. F. L., Blundell, J. E. 1991, 'Food craving, dietary restraint and mood', Appetite, vol. 17, issue 3, pp. 187-197, https://doi.org/10.1016/0195-6663(91)90021-J

Stender, S., Dyerberg, J., & Astrup, A. 2007, 'Fast food: unfriendly and unhealthy', International Journal of Obesity, vol. 31, pp. 887-890, https://doi.org/10.1038/sj.ijo.0803616

Popkess-Vawter, S., Wendel, S., Schmoll, S. & O'Connell Kathleen 1998, 'Overeating, reversal theory, and weight cycling', Western Journal of Nursing Research, vol. 20, issue 1, https://doi.org/10.1177/019394599802000105

Ludwig, D. S., Maizoub, J. A., Al-Zahrani A , Dallal, G. E. , Blanco, I. , Roberts, S. B. 1999, 'High glycemic index foods, overeating, and obesity', Pediatrics, vol.103, issue 3, 10.1542/peds.103.3.e26

Prentice, A. M. 2001, 'Overeating: the health risks', Obesity research, vol. 9, issue S11, pp. 234S-238S, https://doi.org/10.1038/oby.2001.124

Robinson, E., Aveyard, P., Daley, A., Jolly, K., Lewis, A. , Lycett, D., Higgs, S. 2013, 'Eating attentively: a systematic review and meta-analysis of the effect of food intake memory and awareness on eating', The American Journal of Clinical Nutrition, vol. 97, issue 4, pp. 728-742, https://doi.org/10.3945/ajcn.112.045245

Wansink, B., Just, D. R., Payne, C. 2009, 'Mindless eating and healthy heuristics for the irrational', American Economic Review, vol. 99, issue 2, pp. 165-169, 10.1257/aer.99.2.165

Cheung, L., Hanh, T. N. 2010, Savor: mindful eating, mindful life, Harper One, New York.

Tryon, M. S., Carter, C. S., DeCant, R., Laugero, K. D. 2013, 'Chronic stress exposure may affect the brain's response to high calorie food cues and predispose to obesogenic eating habits', Physiology & Behavior, vol. 120, pp. 233-242, https://doi.org/10.1016/j.physbeh.2013.08.010

Ownby, R. L., Acevedo, A., Jacobs, R. J., Caballero, J., Waldrop-Valverde, D. 2014, 'Negative and positive beliefs related to health and mood', American Journal of Health Behavior, vol. 38, issue 4, pp. 586-597, https://doi.org/10.5993/AJHB.38.4.12

Kennedy, A. K., Schneiderman, J. U., Ramseyer Winter V. 2019, 'Association of body weight perception and unhealthy weight control behaviours in adolescence', Children and Youth Services Review, vol. 96, pp. 250-254, https://doi.org/10.1016/j.childyouth.2018.11.053

Jones, J. M., Bennett, S., Olmsted, M. P., Lawson, M. L., Rodin, G. 2001, 'Disordered eating attituded and behaviours in teenaged girls: a school-based study', CMAJ, vol.165, issue 5, pp. 547-552, http://www.cmaj.ca/content/165/5/547.full

Hill, A. J. 2006, 'Motivation for eating behaviour in adolescent girls: the body beautiful', Proceedings of the Nutrition Society, vol. 65, issue 4, pp. 376-384, https://doi.org/10.1079/PNS2006513

Johnson, F., Wardle, J., Griffith, J. 2002, 'The adolescent food habits checklist: reliability and validity of a measure of healthy eating behaviour in adolescents', European Journal of Clinical Nutrition, vol. 56, pp. 644-649, https://www.nature.com/articles/1601371

www.ingramcontent.com/pod-product-compliance
Lightning Source LLC
Chambersburg PA
CBHW051617030426
42334CB00030B/3225